The Essential Lower Back Pain Exercise Guide

Treat Low Back Pain at Home in Just Twenty-One Days

Morgan Sutherland, L.M.T.

The Essential Lower Back Pain Exercise Guide

Copyright © 2018 Morgan Sutherland

Photos: Online images, labeled for reuse

Illustrations: Copyright Morgan Sutherland

Cover image: 123RF

Contents

Medical Disclaimer

The information provided in this book is not intended to be a substitute for professional medical advice, diagnosis, or treatment. Never disregard or delay seeking professional medical advice, because of something you read in this book. Never rely on information in this book in place of seeking professional medical advice.

Morgan Sutherland is not responsible or liable for any advice, course of treatment, diagnosis, other information, services, and/or products that you obtain in this book. You are encouraged to consult with your doctor or healthcare provider with regard to the information contained in this book. After reading this book, you are encouraged to review the information carefully with your professional healthcare provider.

Personal Disclaimer

I am not a doctor. The information I provide is based on my personal experiences and research as a licensed massage therapist. Any recommendations I make about posture, exercise, stretching, and massage should be discussed between you and your professional healthcare provider to prevent any risk to your health.

My Back Pain Story

I never imagined I'd ever get back pain, but it was a scorching hot July day and somebody had to lug that 60-pound Friedrich air conditioner up a flight of stairs. That somebody was me, and I threw my back out in the process.

The pain started as a sharp pain in my left, upper hip region, and when I went to sleep, I felt a burning sensation in my lower spine. It was a horrible beginning to my summer, even though I did have cool air for my family, as a result of my labors.

I had to limp around, and it took everything in me to not walk with a grimace, moaning and groaning in agony. I couldn't stop moving, because my work kept me on my feet all day. It also didn't help that I had a long commute. Instead of being overjoyed by the enthusiastic greetings of my kids when I arrived home, I would dodge their hugs and collapse on the floor in agony.

But what really did me in was taking my family to the beach right after the initial back injury. I dropped them off at the beach entrance with half the beach gear and then parked. I then had to walk about a mile uphill, lugging the remaining beach gear. I could feel my lower back twinge, as I suffered my way up the hill.

Not being the pill-popping type, I refused to take a muscle relaxant. So, instead I took two doses of 200 milligrams of ibuprofen. It didn't make a dent in the pain or help me get a good night's sleep.

My lower back and hip were in bad shape. I needed to take action and get help fast.

As a professional massage therapist, I had witnessed the effectiveness of deep-tissue massage on lower back pain. Unfortunately, I was leery that even a skilled massage therapist could help me relieve the pain, because the therapist has to be extra cautious to avoid massaging directly over the injured muscles. I didn't want to make things worse.

A colleague referred me to a well-known orthopedic acupuncturist, who works with a number of prominent physical therapists.

Regrettably, that didn't do the trick, and I limped away feeling frustrated, because the pain was still there. I started to get nervous.

Dark, depressing thoughts clouded my mind with "what if" scenarios, like what if I've truly damaged my back and won't be able to provide for my family. But I needed to shake these negative thoughts out of my head, if not for me, then for the sake of my wife and kids.

Since the days were longer, we took after-dinner walks at a nearby recreation center, which had a soccer field and a track. My wife power walked away, pushing our two year old in the stroller, as I slowly hobbled at a snail's pace. I felt embarrassed, as if I had aged 30 years, and had stressful thoughts of what if I can't work, what if it's really something that needs surgery. I couldn't see a silver lining.

A dark cloud of despair followed me around the track as I dragged my body—I was a sorry sight. Sitting began bothering me, and walking on hard floors REALLY bothered me. I could feel the pain in my hip joints and hot burning pain at the base of my lower back.

I was living a nightmare and I knew it was time to see my doctor. Miraculously, I was able to get an appointment right away. What he shared with me changed the course of my back pain for the better.

My doctor, who happened to be a doctor of osteopathic medicine (DO), assessed my back and ruled out disc herniation, because there was no leg weakness and sensory loss (phew!). It wasn't sciatica, because there wasn't any radiating pain down my leg. I was diagnosed as having lumbar disc disease, which sounds scary, but in layman terms means nonspecific or mechanical low back pain. My back felt worse with flexion or forward bending and felt better with extension.

He performed a **3-second technique** a couple of times and then asked me to walk across the room. The pain in my left hip had considerably decreased but was still there. He told me that **within a week** or so I should be feeling a lot less pain and recommended a number of stretches and lumbar stabilization/core strengthening exercises.

I took action and practiced all the exercises he recommended at least one to two times per day. Within three weeks of my doctor's visit, I was pain free and my back was stronger.

~~~~~

After my lower back pain had vanished, I made it my mission to share these back-pain relief secrets with my massage clients who suffered from acute and chronic back pain.

I called it *The Essential Lower Back Pain Exercise Guide.*

When back pain strikes, it can ruin your life. Reaching for opiates as a quick fix can be ineffective and even dangerous for your health.

I've done the hard work of finding all the best core strengthening exercises and back pain relief stretches, so you don't need to waste hours scouring the Internet looking for which exercises work best.

Now, if you think you have a herniated disc, then you should consult your doctor first before starting a rehab-style exercise program. But for regular back pain, I have a routine just for you, and if you have sciatica, I also have a specific routine for you.

- You don't need a fancy gym to do these exercises.
- You don't need to trek across town to see a physical therapist two or three times per week.
- You don't need to buy any costly back pain relief machines.
- You don't need to purchase an ergonomic chair or special shoe inserts.
- You don't need to wear a Velcro back belt. Those don't work!

All you need is a mat or comfortable surface (not a bed), such as a rug or carpet, and that's it. There are a few exercise accessories that will set you back about $20. In addition, you need the determination and willpower to do the exercises.

I did them every day for 21 days, and BOOM—my back pain vanished, and I felt stronger and walked faster than I did before. I remember the day when I stopped limping around the track and could actually race my speedy six year old. I had to slow myself down to let him win, and when I stopped, my back felt fine. Fine!

My back pain became just a distant memory, but I had this vibrant enthusiasm to share these exercise routines with anyone I knew who had back pain, so they could obtain the relief that I had.

What I kept coming across with many of my back pain clients was TIME. They said they didn't have the time to do a 15- or 30-minute routine every day. OK, I get that. I made the time for myself with two kids, a busy work week, 90 minutes a day of commuting in the car. Hey, if I can make that time, you can too.

Feeling good, feeling healthy, is important. It's essential that we feel our best to make the most of every day. Let me show you how to do that!

Got Back Pain? Now What?

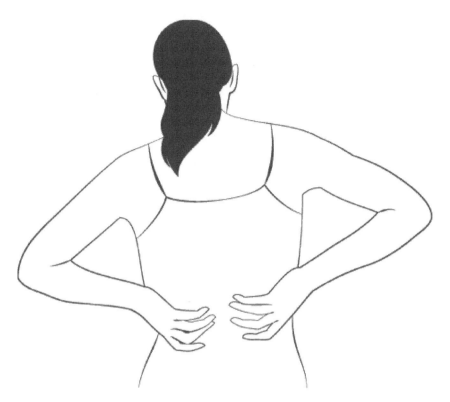

Chronic pain, affecting approximately 100 million people each year, is classified as pain persisting for 12 weeks or more. Low back pain is the most common kind of chronic pain complaint. When the body's pain signals keep firing in the nervous system for this length of time, it can have a draining effect on a person's quality of life—physically, mentally, and spiritually.

In the United States, 8 out of 10 people will experience low back pain at some time in their lives. Low back pain is the second most frequent reason for doctor visits, next to the common cold, and it is the leading cause of job-related disabilities.

When sudden and acute back pain strikes, it can cause intense shooting or stabbing pain that dramatically limits movement. This is often to the point that standing upright can feel like a Sisyphean task—repeatedly rolling the same rock up the hill without any relief. This pain can last anywhere from a few days to weeks.

Subacute back pain, pain lasting 4–12 weeks, is generally the result of a strained or pulled muscle—that's when the muscle or tendon is ripped or torn, from overstretching it, or by pulling the muscle in one direction while it is contracting in the other direction. Muscle strains are typically caused from a fall, careless lifting technique, poor posture, or a sudden movement.

When the muscles are strained or torn, the area around the muscles become inflamed. This inflammation leads to back spasms, and it is the back spasms that can cause both acute low back pain and difficulty moving.

Finding a quick fix for your back pain can be a slippery slope, due to all the back pain myths and misconceptions.

Let's pull back the curtains and reveal the truth about back pain and debunk the nine common back pain myths.

Nine Common Back Pain Myths

1. Bed Rest Is the Best Cure for Back Pain

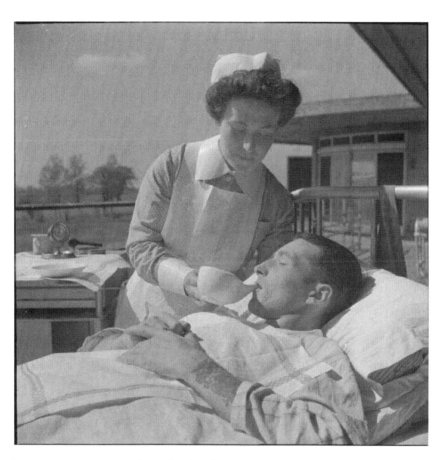

In some cases, going the bed rest route and taking a day or two off from work to "rest your back" can quickly resolve a temporary back strain. One of the main reasons it's recommended is to reduce pressure on the discs in the spine and to stop the mechanical stresses that are irritating pain receptors. A short period of bed rest might help reduce acute back pain.

However, prolonged immobilization can have adverse effects, such as depression, blood clots in the legs, muscle atrophy, or even muscle splinting (when the muscle becomes extremely tight and contracted).

In fact, a 1996 Finnish study found that people who, following the onset of lower back pain, kept moving without bed rest had better back flexibility than those who rested in bed for a week.

2. Really Bad Back Pain Can Lead to Paralysis

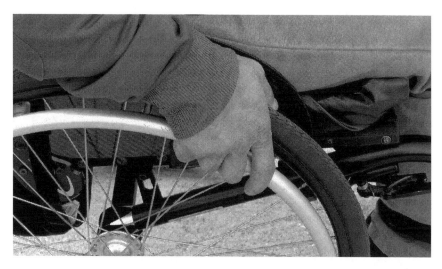

The spinal cord ends in the upper part of the low back (lumbar 1). At the base of the low back (lumbar 4 and 5), there are only nerve roots, which are extremely tough structures. By and large, a lot of back pain does not usually point toward a back problem that could bring about paralysis. A few examples of extraordinary cases where paralysis might be a risk include spine tumors, spinal infections, and unstable spine fractures.

See http://www.spine-health.com/conditions/lower-back-pain/myths-and-reality-back-pain-and-back-problems

3. The Severity of Back Pain Is Linked to the Severity of Back Damage

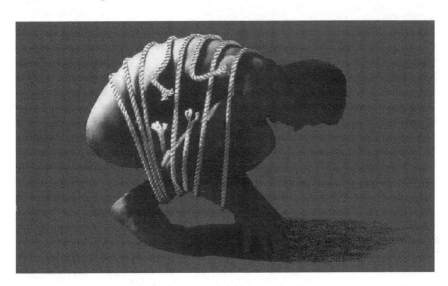

With acute pain, the level of pain is linked to the level of damage (for example, if you touch a hot iron, you will immediately feel a great deal of pain). However, with chronic back pain (longer than six weeks), the amount of pain isn't usually connected to the amount of damage.

4. One of My Parents Had a Bad Back, So, I'll Probably Have One Too

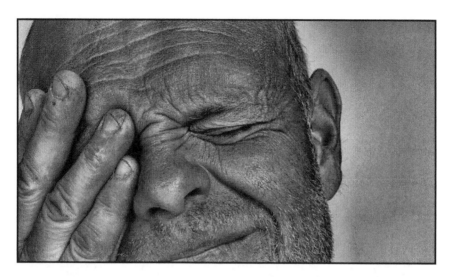

For the vast majority of conditions related to back pain, there is no genetic predisposition, which means that parents do not pass their back conditions to their children.

5. An MRI Scan Will Reveal Exactly What's Wrong with My Back

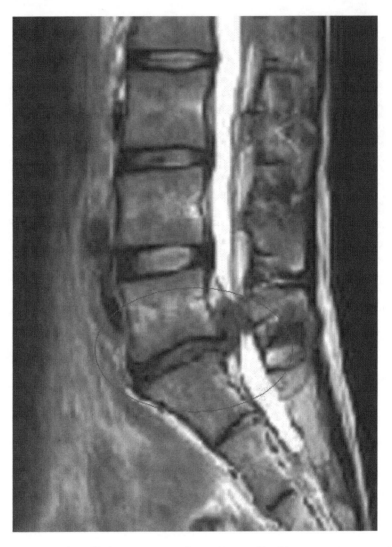

Sometimes it will, but more often, it won't. Also, even people without back pain can have changes in their spine, so magnetic resonance imaging (MRI) scans can make a person more anxious and fearful than they need to be, making the problem worse.

More often than not, an MRI scan is used when patients are not responding to appropriate back pain treatment.

An abnormality that is seen on an imaging test (MRI, computers tomography or CT scan) does not necessarily cause back pain. In fact, the majority of people who never have had low back pain will have abnormalities (such as a herniated disc or degenerative disc) on an imaging test. For patients experiencing low back pain, 92–96 percent can be treated successfully without back surgery.

6. NSAIDs Are a Good Choice for Dealing with Back Pain

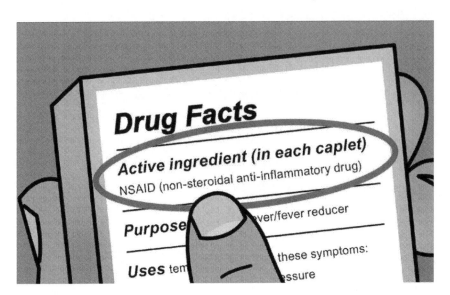

Taking non-steroidal anti-inflammatory drugs (NSAIDs), such as ibuprofen and naproxen, can lead to accidental overdose. Prolonged use can be dangerous for a person's cardiovascular health, carrying severe side effects, such as gastrointestinal and kidney damage.

According to data from the US federal government, acetaminophen, the active ingredient in Tylenol, can lead to liver failure and kills more than 150 Americans each year after accidentally taking too much. So, if and when that low back pain hits, you might want to think twice about taking a double dose.

7. Surgery Is the Only Real Option That Will Correct the Problem That Is Causing Back Pain

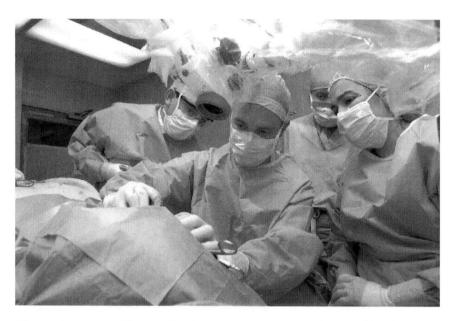

Close to one million spinal surgeries are performed in the United States each year. One quarter of them are spinal fusions, costing about $60,000 each. Most of these surgeries have a low success rate and usually require re-operation. A majority of surgery patients are left in pain, out of work, and dependent on pain-relieving drugs.

8. Injections Are a Safe Option for Relieving Back Pain

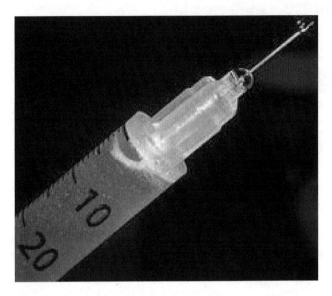

Many pain sufferers try steroid injections to ease their discomfort, but researchers now say this quick fix provides only modest, short-term relief. In fact, it was found that a single steroid injection eased pain for one month, and after that, the effectiveness faded.

Steroid shots are used primarily for their anti-inflammatory effects. It is usually only indicated if there are signs of radiculopathy (nerve impingement with symptoms going down the leg).

While topical steroids can cause skin thinning, the concern with injections is the absorption of the steroid which can affect one's own production of steroid hormones, as well as weakening of the tissue in the surrounding area of the injection (if patients are given too many injections), making the person more susceptible to further injury.

9. Exercise Is Bad for Back Pain

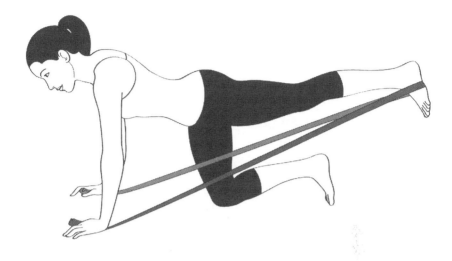

Regular exercise *prevents* back pain. And doctors might recommend exercise for people who have recently hurt their lower backs. The doctors will usually suggest that the person start with gentle movements and gradually build up the intensity. Once the immediate pain goes away, an exercise plan can help keep it from coming back.

The National Institute of Neurological Disorders and Stroke (NINDS) says on its website that, *"Exercise may be the most effective way to speed recovery from low back pain and help strengthen back and abdominal muscles. . . . Maintaining and building muscle strength is particularly important for persons with skeletal irregularities."*

According to health researcher Chris Maher at the University of Sydney in Australia, after analyzing 21 global studies (involving more than 30,000 participants) on how to treat and prevent lower back pain, those who use a combination of exercise and back pain education reduced the risk of repeated low back pain in the year following an episode between 25 and 40 percent. It didn't really matter what kind of exercise—core strengthening, aerobic exercise, or flexibility and stretching.

"What we do understand about the back is that the more you use it, the more likely you are to keep it strong, fit and healthy," says Maher.

See http://www.npr.org/sections/health-shots/2016/01/11/462366361/forget-the-gizmos-exercise-works-best-for-lower-back-pain

Before we get into the specific back pain exercise routine that helped fix my back pain problem, let's look at the four most common causes of back pain.

Four Most Common Causes of Back Pain

Neglected postures, such as rounding your low back while sitting for extended periods of time in front of the computer, standing for hours stooped over, sleeping improperly, and lifting poorly, can all lead to chronic back pain.

Maintaining the natural lumbar curve in your low back is essential to preventing posture-related back pain. This natural curve works as a shock absorber, helping to distribute weight along the length of your spine.

Below are the four most common causes of back pain:

#1 Postural Neglect

- Rounding your low back while sitting for extended hours in front of the computer

- Poor lifting techniques

- Prolonged forward bending while working

- Standing or lying for long periods of time in a poor position

#2 Sitting

- Slouching while sitting at a restaurant, café, or movie theater

- Sedentary office jobs that require endless hours of sitting can overstretch the back muscles, distorting the vertebrae, potentially causing bulging or herniated discs

#3 Standing (or Poor Lying Posture)

- Standing (or lying) for long periods of time, the lordosis can become excessive and pain results

- Working in stooped positions when doing yard work or household chores, such as raking, shoveling, or vacuuming

#4 Lifting

- Lifting objects with a rounded back can put unwanted pressure on the vertebral discs. Keeping the body upright, avoiding back flexion, and maintaining a natural lordotic curve is a better option when lifting.

Source: *Treat Your Own Back*

Prolonged Sitting and Back Pain

In today's culture, everyone's constantly plugged into some device, be it a computer, laptop, tablet, or smartphone. Sedentary lifestyles inevitably result in clocking thousands of hours with our bodies resembling a human question mark—our heads jutting forward, our shoulders rounding, and our stomachs getting closer to our knees.

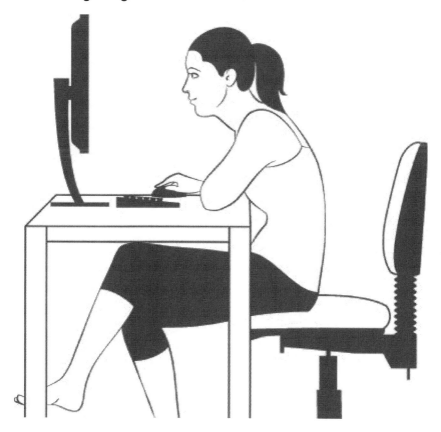

Sitting for too long causes your low back muscles and hip flexors (the muscles that allow you to lift your knees and bend at your waist) to become short and tight. Slumped over in a chair all day also makes your abdominal muscles slowly lose tone and your glutes (also known as the buttocks) to become overstretched and weak.

Another phenomenon that happens with prolonged sitting is that it causes an anterior (or front) tilt, which is an adaptive shortening of the hip flexor muscles. When moving from a prolonged sitting position to an upright one, the shortened hip flexors inevitably pull on the muscle attachments of the lumbar (low back) spine, causing an anterior shift in the hips. This can put unwanted strain on the low back, exaggerate the lumbar curve, and potentially cause a bulging or herniated disc.

Sit the Right Way

If you have to sit for extended periods of time, maintaining good posture is key! Chronic slouching or leaning to one side, even if these positions make the pain subside, are bad habits that propagate back pain.

The National Institute of Neurological Disorders and Stroke recommends sitting in a chair with good low back support. If sitting for a long time, you should rest your feet on a low stool. If possible, switch sitting positions and get up and walk around a bit throughout the day.

Reprogram Your Body to Sit Correctly in Eight Moves

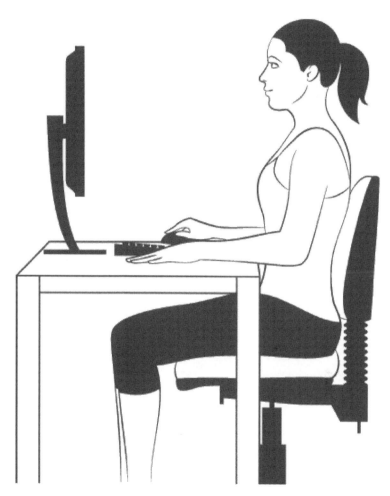

1. Sit back in your chair. If you can't sit back, support your low back with a lumbar roll, rolled towel, or small pillow.

2. Don't lean forward and sit on the edge of your chair. This will cause your low back to arch, your head to drop forward, and your shoulders to round.

3. Drop your shoulders and keep them relaxed, so it doesn't look like you're wearing them as earrings.

4. Keep your arms close to your sides.

5. Make sure your elbows are bent 90 degrees.

6. Stretch the top of your head toward the ceiling, and tuck your chin in slightly.

7. Keep your upper back and neck comfortably straight by rolling your shoulders back and tucking in your tummy about 20 percent.

8. Place your feet flat on the floor, pointing them forward so your knees are level with your hips. If necessary, prop up your feet with a footstool or other support.

Two Accessories That Will Help Improve Your Sitting Posture and Take Pressure Off Your Lower Back

1. McKenzie Lumbar Roll

These back supports are ideal in the car, at the office, or for use with any seat that does not provide adequate lumbar support. They help ensure proper spine alignment and posture while sitting, providing comfortable back pain relief for the lumbar (low back) region.

2. Coccyx Orthopedic Memory Foam Seat Cushion

Flat, hard, and even traditionally padded seating surfaces cause pressure on your coccyx (tailbone).

This causes—

- Poor posture
- Improper spine alignment
- Decreased blood circulation
- Pinched nerves

The Xtreme Comforts Ortho-Seat is ergonomically designed with a coccyx comfort space to help eliminate back pain by reducing focused body weight pressure on the tailbone.

The contour distributes body weight across the seat, relieving pressure while allowing your tailbone to "float" in the open space, not compressed against the seating surface bearing the weight of your body.

See the Reference section for links to order these two accessories.

Get Up, Stand Up

Sometimes you can't avoid stooping. When you are doing yard work or household chores that require you to bend over, make sure to keep your knees bent and your back straight.

Lifting objects with a rounded back can put unwanted pressure on the vertebral discs (bones in the spinal column) and potentially injure your low back. Keeping the body upright, maintaining a natural lumbar curve, is a better option when lifting.

According to the American Academy of Orthopaedic Surgeons, if you are going to lift something:

- Position yourself as close to the object as possible, so that you are more stable.

- Keep your feet shoulder width apart to create a solid base of support.

- Always bend at the knees, tighten your abdominals, and lift with your legs.

When you stand for long periods of time, your lumbar curve can become excessive, and pain can result (this is called lordosis). The illustration below is a perfect example of a person with poor standing posture. You've probably seen someone like this, waiting to place her order at your favorite coffee shop, with her head stooped over her phone like the hunchback Quasimodo.

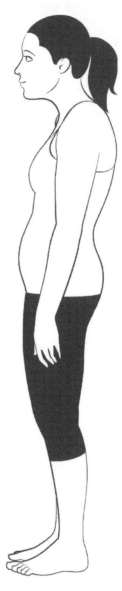

You'll notice the shoulders are rounded, causing the upper back muscles to overstretch and tighten the chest muscles. This posture can potentially compress the brachial plexus, which is the network of nerves that originate in the neck and feed into the armpit region and down into the arms. A brachial plexus impingement can lead to a number of problems, from numbness in the hands, to thoracic outlet syndrome or carpal tunnel-like symptoms. In this hunched posture, the abdominals are loose, which gives them an exaggerated lumbar curve.

This kind of slouched posture can trigger low back pain, neck pain, headaches, tendonitis, and also lead to worn-out, imbalanced muscles. It's like an energy vampire, sucking away any vibrant spirit you possess.

I'm going to show you how to combat this slouched posture in six moves.

How to Stand the Right Way in Six Moves

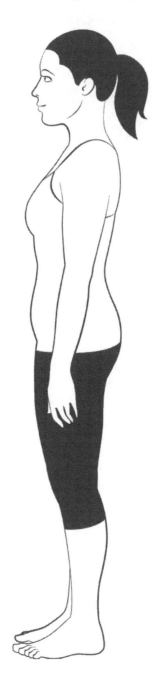

Good posture allows your spine to be aligned and balanced. You can breathe deeply, because your lungs and diaphragm have more space to expand and contract. Not only will you feel more energized and less worn down, but you'll also look good and be twice as likely to smile.

1. First, stand with your feet pointing forward or slightly turned inward.

2. Now, squeeze your glutes tightly and rotate your feet inward, so that your big toes slightly turn toward each other.

3. Tighten your thighs, about 50 percent.

4. Slightly tighten your abdominals, only about 20 percent.

5. Now, roll your shoulders back. This brings your shoulder blades closer together and your chest moves up and forward.

6. Last, turn your hands so that your thumbs are facing forward.

Voila! Your now have perfect standing posture.

So, now that you are equipped with this perfect sitting and standing posture advice, we can get to the twenty-one back pain relief exercise routine.

Twenty-One Day, Low Back Pain, Relief Program

How to Use This Book

Twenty-One Exercises, Thirty Minutes or Less/Day

For the best results, do the twenty-one exercises every day for twenty-one days.

If that's not feasible, do the flexibility exercises five days per week and the core strengthening exercises three to four times per week.

Sitting for long periods of time, puts the quadriceps muscles (thighs) in a constant contraction, keeping them short and tight.

Of the four quadriceps muscles, only one of them, the rectus femoris, attaches at the hip near the knee.

Tight quadriceps pull the pelvis forward at the front part of your hips, called the anterior superior iliac spine (ASIS). This pulling tilts the pelvis downward or forward, resulting in what's called an anterior pelvic tilt.

This anterior tilt increases the arch in the lower back (referred to as lordosis), and this can make the back muscles tight and sore. Inadvertently, the tight quads can weaken or overstretch the hamstrings.

Good postural alignment, stretched out quads, and strong hamstrings will help to balance and protect the low back muscles and keep them pain free.

Ten Stretches and Eleven Core and Back-Strengthening Exercises

For the first exercise, you're going to stretch your quads.

1a. Quadriceps Lying Down Stretch (Contract-Relax Version)

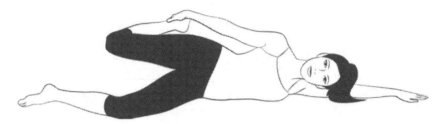

Lie on your side and contract your abdominals, before grasping the top of your foot to bring your ankle toward your glutes. Hold stretch for 10 seconds and then for 6 seconds; attempt to straighten your leg, but let your hands "win." Then relax and stretch your heel toward your glutes for 30 seconds.

Turn to your other side and repeat on the opposite leg.

1b. Couch Potato Quad Stretch

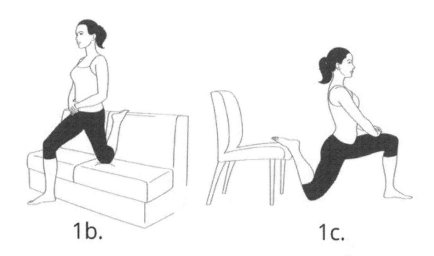

1b.   1c.

Start by placing your left knee on to the couch cushion with your left foot against the back of the couch. The closer your knee is to the back cushion, the more intense a stretch it will be; the farther from the back cushion, the easier it is.

If this is too painful for the top of your foot, place a rolled-up towel or small pillow underneath that foot/ankle.

Once you've gotten into this position, SLOWLY bring the right leg into a lunge, making sure that the knee is over the ankle and not past the toes.

From here, kick your left foot into the back cushion to contract (resist) the muscles on the front of the leg (quadriceps).

As you kick into the back cushion, use your other leg to push your body back to stretch the quads. As you go back, be sure to tuck the glutes under (the opposite of sticking your butt out) in order to increase the stretch.

Move back and forth for 1 minute. Then repeat on the other leg.

1c. Couch Potato Quad Stretch (version 2)

If no couch is available, a chair will do the trick.

See https://premiersportsandspine.com/2015/06/the-best-stretch-for-your-hip-flexors-the-couch-stretch/

2a. Hip Flexor Stretch

Did you know that a tight psoas could be causing your back pain?

The psoas muscle is a major hip flexor, located deep in the abdominal contents and spans from the upper portion of the femur to the lumbar vertebrae. It affects your posture and helps to stabilize your spine.

The psoas enables you to walk and run. Every time you lift your knee, it contracts. When your leg swings back, the psoas lengthens.

The psoas often gets short from too much sitting. If your psoas is tight and in a contracted state, it will bring your lower back forward, moving you into an anterior tilt: creating a lordotic curve. This pressure can ultimately compress the joints and discs of the lumbar vertebrae and cause degeneration, which will make them more susceptible to injury.

So regularly stretching your psoas can help prevent future injuries from occurring, or it can mend a chronically tight psoas.

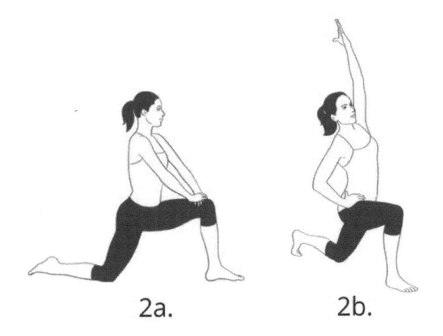

2a.   2b.

To effectively stretch the hip flexors, first kneel on your right knee, with toes down, and place your left foot flat on the floor in front of you.

Place both hands on your left thigh and press your hips forward until you feel a good stretch in the hip flexors.

Contract your abdominals and slightly tilt your pelvis back, while keeping your chin parallel to the floor. Hold this pose for 20 to 30 seconds, and then switch sides.

2b. Hip Flexor Stretch
(with Arm Raised over Head)

First, kneel onto your right knee, with toes down, and place your left foot flat on the floor in front of you.

Place both hands on your left thigh and press your hips forward until you feel a good stretch in the hip flexors.

Reach your hands over your head and arch your body back.

Contract your abdominals and slightly tilt your pelvis back while keeping your chin parallel to the floor. Hold this pose for 30 seconds, and then switch sides. Stretch your non-dominant side first.

Source: *The Four-Hour Body*, p. 352.

3. Adductor Stretches

The inner thigh muscles, known as the adductors, play a crucial role in movement and stabilization of the legs and pelvis. The adductors help support the pelvis and allow you to bring your legs toward and across the midline of your body. Tight adductors can distort the posture and accentuate the anterior tilt, which contributes to low back pain. Weak adductors can throw off a person's gait and force the body to compensate so as to maintain pelvic stability.

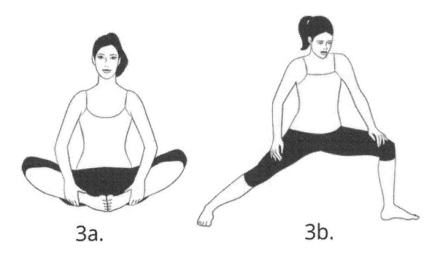

3a. 3b.

3a. Butterfly Stretch

The butterfly stretch is a static stretch that helps to improve the flexibility of your adductors.

First, sit on the floor or a mat, open your hips, flex your knees, and move your feet together. Grasp your ankles and gently pull them up, as you simultaneously push your elbows into your knees. Hold for 30 seconds.

3b. Sideways Lunge Adductor Stretch

If you prefer to do this adductor stretch standing, then the sideways lunge is for you. Keep the rear foot sideways and flat on the floor, and bend the front leg gently, until you feel a gentle stretch along the inside of your leg.

Keep your body upright—there is no need to lean forward. Hold this stretch for 30 seconds, and then repeat with your other leg.

4. Hamstring Stretches

Desk jockeys who sit all day long are guaranteed to have tight hamstrings. These are the group of muscles that help bend your knee and extend your hips. They are located on the back of your upper thigh.

When the hamstrings are too tight, they can pull the backside of the pelvis downward. This downward pull of the pelvis can cause a flattening of your back, which increases pressure on the bones of your lumbar spine.

If this pulling happens for an extended time period, it causes the muscles in the low back, which hold your body upright, to become weak and start to fatigue, as they try to hold your body upright against gravity. For this reason, stretching the hamstrings is crucial to help reduce the strain on your low back.

4a. Static Hamstring Stretch (Lying Down)

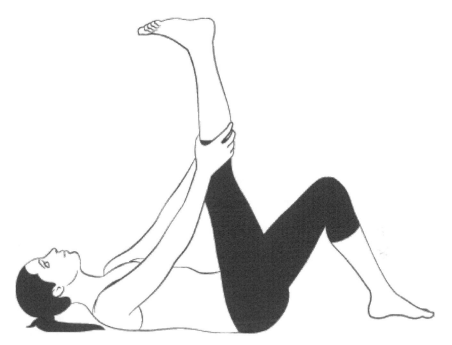

Grab the back of your leg with both hands. Pull your leg toward you gently, while keeping both hips on the floor.

Hold for 30 seconds. Contract your abdominals when bringing your legs up. Repeat on the other leg.

4b. Hamstring Stretch with Yoga Strap
(Contract-Relax)

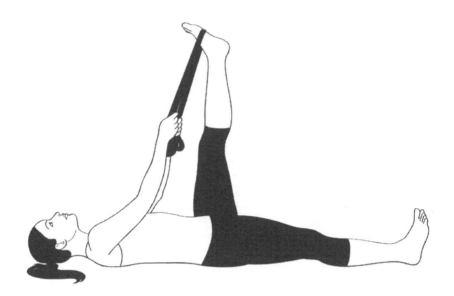

Using a yoga strap or stretch strap has been shown to be extremely effective at increasing the hamstring's flexibility and restoring range of motion.

To perform a proprioceptive neuromuscular facilitation (PNF) hamstring stretch (contract-relax antagonist-contract) using a strap, lie on your back and loop the strap around the ball of your foot, holding the ends of the strap with both hands.

Try to keep your chin down and your shoulders back. Exhale, while pushing your heel up toward the ceiling. Hold this stretch for 20 to 30 seconds. Keeping your knee straight, push down with your heel into the strap toward the floor for 3 to 5 seconds. Then try to straighten your knee and actively push your foot up toward the ceiling, contracting your quadriceps. Hold this for 3 to 5 seconds.

Relax and then hold this stretch for 20 to 30 seconds. Repeat on the other leg.

See http://www.stretching-exercises-guide.com/hamstring-stretches.html

5. IT Band Stretch with Yoga Strap

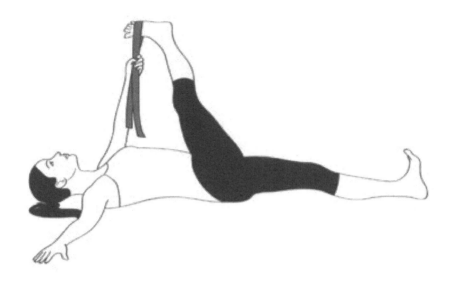

Illiotibial band syndrome (ITBS) is a common injury. The IT band is connective tissue that runs parallel to the femur from the hip to the knee.

Keep your leg straight, raise it, and slowly drop it across your body.

Keep your hips down, and let that leg drop over. You should feel that stretch all the way through the outside of your leg.

Hold the stretch for 30 seconds, and then repeat on the other leg.

6. Piriformis Stretch

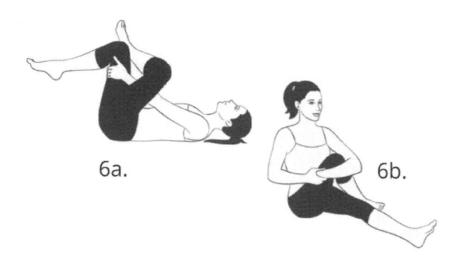

6a.   6b.

6a. Piriformis Stretch (Lying Down)

The piriformis is a tiny, pear-shaped muscle deep in the glutes that helps laterally rotate the hip. If gets too tight, it can impinge the sciatica nerve that runs through or under it, causing tremendous pain, tingling, and numbness through the glutes and into the lower leg. This condition is called piriformis syndrome.

When performing the piriformis stretch, make sure to contract your abdominals before crossing your leg and resting your foot on the other knee. Hold this stretch for 30 seconds, and then repeat with your other leg.

6b. Piriformis/ Glute Stretch (Sitting)

While in a sitting position, cross your right leg over your straightened left leg. Hug your right knee with your left arm, making sure to keep your back straight.

Hold this stretch for 30 to 60 seconds, and then repeat on the opposite side.

7. Spinal Rotation and Twist

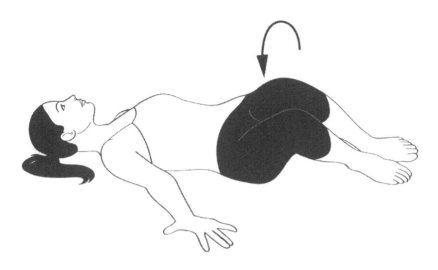

Lie on your back with your feet flat on the floor and gently drop your knees side to side. Draw in your abdominal muscles, like a vacuum, and maintain this contraction throughout the exercise.

Slowly rotate your knees to the right, making sure to keep your hips in contact with the floor. Engage your lateral abdominals (obliques) to help you pull your knees back to the center, and then repeat on the opposite side. Repeat 10–20 times.

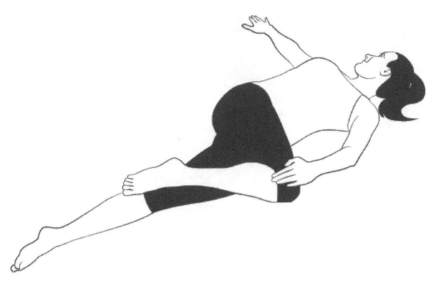

Remain on the floor and stretch both legs out. With your right arm stretched to the right, lift your right knee across your left knee. Contract your abdominals before bringing your knee up and over the leg. Hold for 20 seconds. Repeat this move with the other knee.

8. Cat and Cow Pose

Starting on your hands and knees, move into the Cat Pose by slowly pressing your spine up, arching your back.

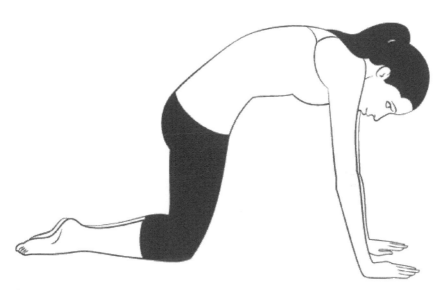

Hold the pose for a few seconds, and then move to the Cow Pose by scooping your spine in, pressing your shoulder blades back and lifting your head.

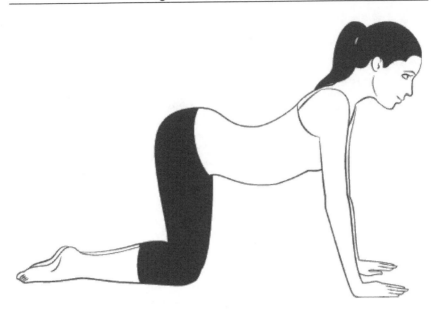

Moving back and forth from Cat Pose to Cow Pose helps move your spine to a neutral position, relaxing the muscles and easing tension.

Repeat the sequence 10 times, flowing smoothly from cat to cow, and cow back to cat.

9. Static Extension Position on Elbows

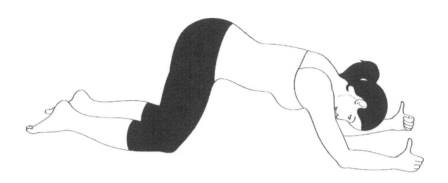

Get on your hands and knees, and make sure your shoulders, elbows, and wrists are aligned in a straight line with your hips directly above your knees.

Next, move your hands a few inches forward making a loose fist with your thumbs up.

Arch your low back by pushing your hips backwards toward your heels.

Let your head drop. Hold this position for 60 seconds.

10. Press Up

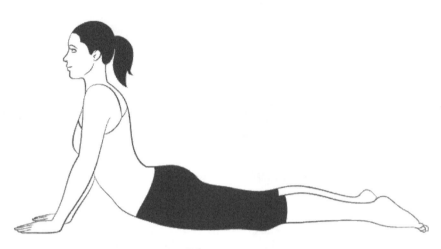

Press your palms into the floor and lift your upper body, keeping hips and pelvis rooted to the floor. Extend through the spine from the tailbone to the neck, allowing your back to arch.

Hold for 2 seconds, and then slowly lower to the start position for one rep. Do 10 reps.

Build a Strong Core

Sedentary lifestyles usually go hand in hand with being unfit and overweight. According to a study published in the *American Journal of Epidemiology*, obese people have a higher prevalence of low back pain than non-overweight individuals do.

Another study, published in the *Arthritis & Rheumatology* journal, reported that overweight and obese adults are more likely to have disc degeneration in their low back than normal-weight adults are. An excessive anterior tilt in the pelvis, coupled with weak abdominal muscles creates an excessive amount of tension in a person's low back. This leads to back pain and the increased likelihood of disc deterioration.

So, it's no secret. If your back is sore and achy, you need to strengthen your core, the abdominal and pelvic muscles that encircle and support the spine.

The "core" consists of specific muscles, which stabilize the spine and pelvis, and run the entire length of the torso. The core muscles make it possible to stand upright, shift your body weight, transfer your energy, and move in any direction.

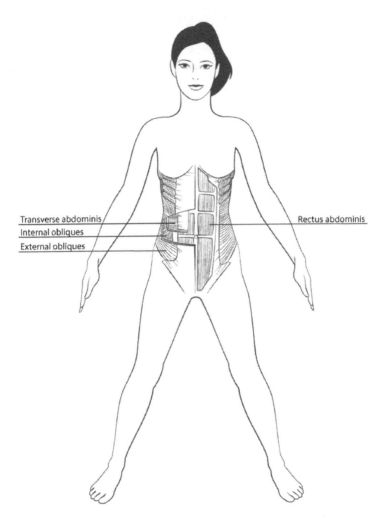

There are four major core muscles: the rectus abdominus, external and internal obliques, and the transverse obliques.

The rectus abdominus extends along the front of the abdomen and forms the "six-pack" muscles.

The external obliques are on the side and front of the abdomen, around your waist.

Underneath the external obliques are the internal obliques. Underneath the internal obliques is the transverse abdominus, which wraps around your spine for protection and stability.

Muscles function with an agonist/antagonist response, so if one muscle takes the brunt of the work, the neglected muscle becomes weakened. Weak core muscles diminish a person's natural lumbar curve, creating a scenario for crippling back pain. A strong, balanced core helps maintain appropriate posture and reduces strain on the spine.

Begin with Pelvic Tilt Warm-Up Exercises

11. Abdominal Draw In (aka Pelvic Tilt)

Lie on your back with your knees bent and feet flat on the floor. In this relaxed position, the small of your back will not be touching the floor.

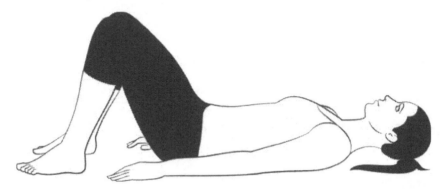

Take a deep breath and on the exhale, pull your abdominals in and push your low back toward the floor. Repeat 20 times.

12. Abdominal Draw In with Knee to Chest

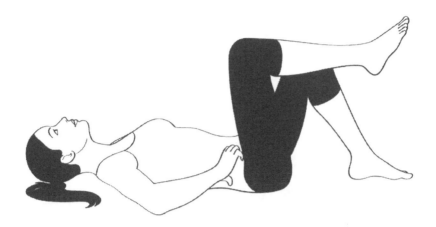

Lie on your back and draw one knee to the chest, while maintaining the abdominal draw in; do not grab the knee with your hand. Repeat 10–20 times with each leg.

13. Abdominal Draw In with Double Knee to Chest

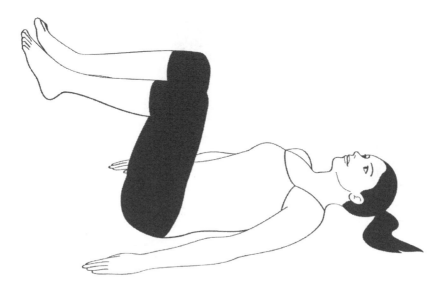

Bring both knees to your chest at the same time. Maintain the abdominal draw in throughout the entire exercise. Repeat 10–20 times.

14. Cat Vomit Exercise
(aka Five Steps to a Flat Belly)

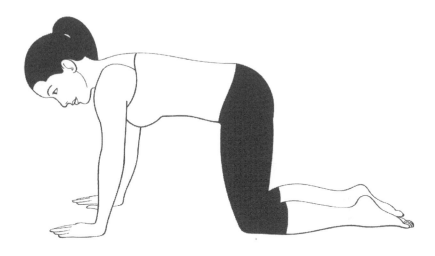

In life-hacking author Tim Ferris's book, *The Four-Hour Body*, he talks about building six-pack abs; the number one muscle you want to target is the deepest one, called the transverse abdominis (TA).

Whenever you do a hard belly laugh or want to get someone's attention by giving an "ahem" cough, that's the TA working.

It's situated right below the rectus abdominis, and it's vital to core and back health, because it literally pulls in what would otherwise be a protruding abdomen. This is why it's nicknamed the "corset muscle."

Step 1

Begin with the all-fours position, without arching your back or straining your neck.

Step 2

Vigorously exhale from your mouth until no more air comes out. You need to fully exhale in order to contract the transverse abdominals, and gravity will provide the resistance.

Step 3

Next, do the vacuum exercise by bringing your belly button upwards toward your spine as hard as you can for 8–12 seconds.

Step 4

As soon you're finished with the 8–12 second hold, fully inhale through the nose.

Step 5

The final step is to take one breath cycle of rest, where you slowly exhale out of your mouth and inhale through the nose.

Repeat the above for a total of 10 repetitions.

15. The Plank

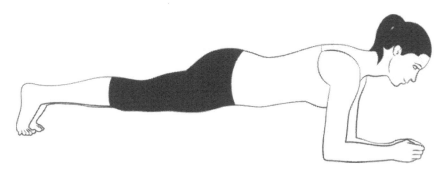

Get into a plank position on the floor with feet hip-width apart and elbows directly under your shoulders.

Brace your core by contracting your abs and attempt to bring your belly button toward your spine.

Keep your back straight and legs and glutes engaged the entire time. Hold this pose for 1 minute.

If 15–30 seconds is all you can do, that's fine, just stay at it. The plank exercise works the transverse abdominis and this helps you sit up straight, hold your shoulders back, and prevent forward head posture.

You might feel sore, but stay at it. In time you'll be able to work your way up to 1 minute.

15a. Front Plank with Alternating Arm Raise (Advanced)

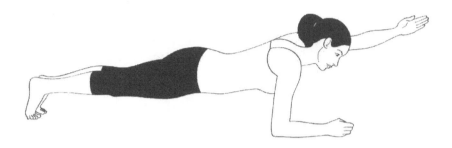

While in the front plank, engage your abs, and extend your left arm in front of you. Hold for 2 seconds and then alternate arms. Repeat 10–15 times each side.

The rocking movement of your body as you shift arms shifts the load to your core muscles, which in turn have to work harder to maintain your balance.

Tip: Keep your head up, eyes forward, and knees straight.

15b. Plank with Hip Extension (Advanced)

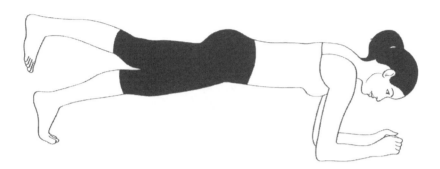

Once you can accomplish 30–45 seconds in a neutral plank position, try to introduce hip extension.

When doing the plank with single leg hip extension, rise, so that you are resting on your forearms and toes. Maintain the abdominal draw in; your back should be completely straight. Now extend your hip/leg upwards and hold for 2 seconds, one leg at a time. Alternate legs. Repeat 10–15 times each side.

16. The Side Plank

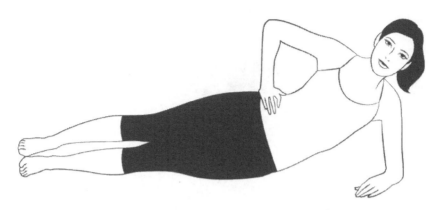

When performing the side plank, start by lying on your side with your forearm on the floor under your shoulder to prop you up, and then stack your feet on top of each other.

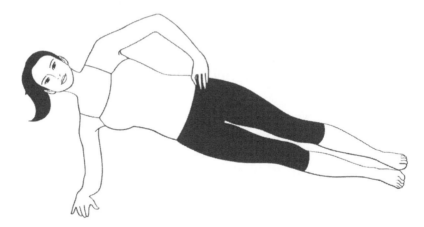

Contract your abdominals and press your forearm into the floor to raise your hips, so that your body is straight from your ankles to your shoulders.

Hold this position for 30–60 seconds, and then repeat on the other side.

Modified Side Plank

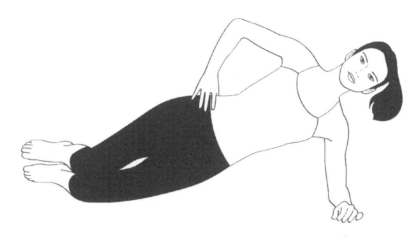

Lie on your left side with your knees bent 90 degrees.

Prop your upper body on your left elbow.

Advanced version: Perform six, 10-second holds on each side (do all your holds on one side, and then switch sides). Rest for 20 seconds, and then perform four, 10-second holds on each side. Rest for 20 seconds, and then perform three, 10-second holds on each side

16a. Side Plank with Hip Abduction (Advanced)

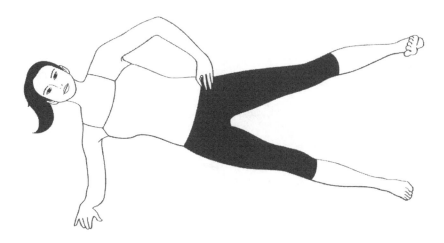

Take this side plank exercise to the next level and raise the upper leg away from the lower leg, abducting the hip.

Hold for 10–20 seconds. Repeat on the other side.

Tip: Don't allow your hips to drop. Maintain a straight line from your shoulders to your ankles.

To modify this exercise, you can bend your bottom leg to 45 degrees and use hand support as needed before moving to the straight leg version.

17. Adductor Assisted Back Extension

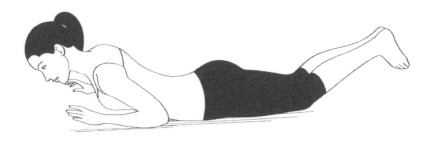

This back extension with raised and squeezed legs works the adductor muscles inside your thighs. The adductors originate in the pelvis and attach to the knee. Contracting these muscles pulls the pelvis down and alleviates compression of the lower spine.

Start by lying flat on your stomach with palms on the floor by your shoulders. Pull your elbows back against your rib cage and your arms up off the ground. Bring your feet and knees firmly together.

Then bend your knees at a 45-degree angle while pressing your knees and feet together as tightly as possible. Lower your feet until they are 6 inches off the ground. Lift your chest as high as you can, while you continue to hold your feet off the ground. Hold the pose for 10–15 seconds. Drop down and then repeat for another 10–15 seconds.

See https://www.youtube.com/watch?v=mZr5ywYLSwQ

Source: *Foundation,* Eric Goodman, pp. 96–97

18. Alternating Superman
(or Superwoman) Exercise

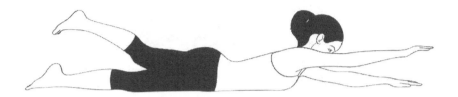

This exercise strengthens the erector spinae back muscles.

Lie face down on the floor on your stomach with arms and legs extended and your neck in a neutral position.

Lift opposite arm and leg for 3–5 seconds and then repeat 10–20 times. Repeat with the opposite arm and leg.

After you're done, you might feel a little achy in the lower back, so just do a quick **Child's Pose** to stretch it out.

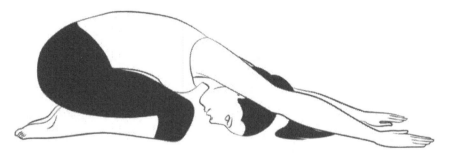

Start with the all-fours position with your arms stretched out straight in front of you, then sit back so your glutes come to rest just above—but not touching—your heels.

Hold the position for 20–30 seconds.

19. Bird Dog (Kneeling Superman)

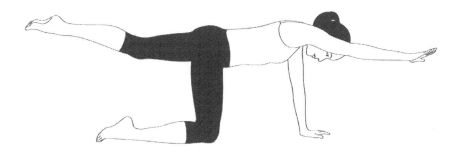

Start with the all-fours position, tighten your hamstrings, glutes, and low back and lift to straighten your leg and opposite arm, while maintaining proper alignment. Make sure to push through your heel.

Hold for 5 seconds. Repeat 6–10 times per side. If you need to modify this exercise, you can focus on extending your legs, one at a time, and not extend your arms.

20. Active Bridge with Knee Pillow Squeeze

One of the major causes of back pain is a weak posterior chain (glutes and hamstrings). The muscles in the front of the body—like the hip flexors and the quadriceps (the anterior kinetic chain)—tend to be stronger, tighter, and shorter than muscles in the back of the body. Sedentary lifestyle, coupled with poor sitting posture, can cause these muscle imbalances.

Bridge exercises reduce back pain by strengthening the glutes and hamstrings and evening out this muscle imbalance.

See http://backpainsolutionsonline.com/announcements-and-releases/backpain/lower-back-pain-causes/weak-posterior-kinetic-chain-cause-of-lower-back-pain

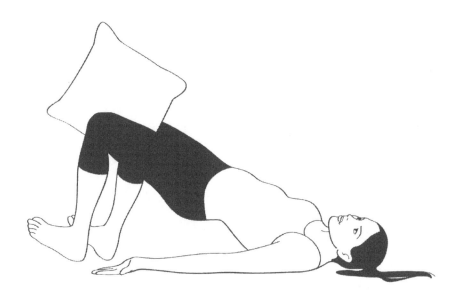

Lie on your back with your knees bent to 90 degrees, aligned with your hips, with a pillow or ball squeezed between your knees.

Press heels into the ground and lift your hips as high as you can, and then slowly lower them. Try to make this a smooth, continuous movement. Repeat 15 times. Do three sets.

21. Bridge with Single Leg Butt Lift

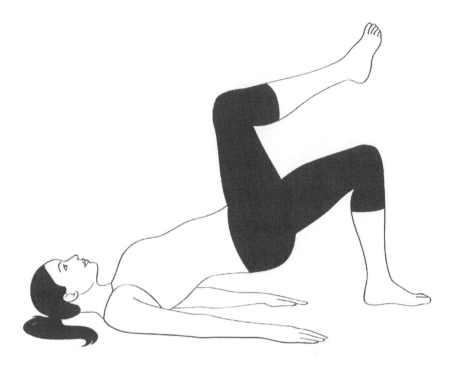

Slowly raise your butt off the floor by using your glutes and hamstrings until your torso is in line with your thighs. Hold for 3–5 seconds. Repeat 10–20 times on each leg.

Finish with Knees to Chest Stretch

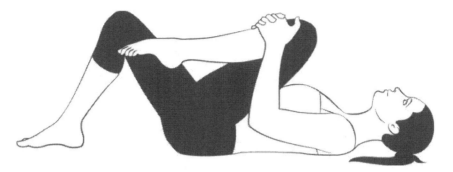

While you're still on your back, with your knees bent, grasp your left knee and pull it to your chest. Hold for 20 seconds.

With your abdominals contracted, try to straighten your right leg. If you experience any discomfort in your back, leave your right leg bent. Repeat this move with the other leg.

Bonus Move: Static Back

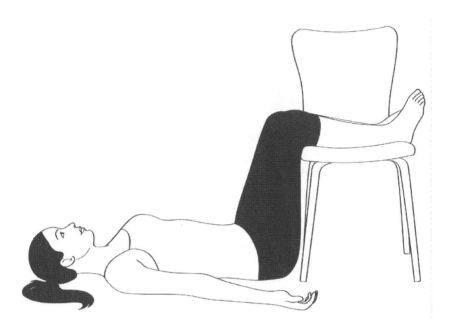

Lie on the floor with your legs resting on a chair. Rest your arms at your side at a 45-degree angle with palms up.

Take deep breaths and let your upper body relax and the curve of your lower back flatten to the floor.

Hold this position for 5 minutes.

The static back position allows gravity to work to begin the balancing process. When you lie on your back and put your legs up on a block or chair, it causes a symmetrical, right-angle posture at the knee joint.

The static back position also causes the pelvis to rotate to a right angle. When that happens, the muscles of the back become bilaterally engaged.

You see, the back muscles can work unilaterally or bilaterally. When you're sitting for long periods in a day, you tend to contort your body, like a question mark, and oftentimes the back muscles on one side of your spine end up working harder than the muscles on the other side. This is not ideal for creating a balanced, pain-free back. This is why the static back position is very effective for creating a balanced back after a long day.

Fifteen-Minute, Doctor-Recommended, Back Pain Relief Exercise Routine

This is the exact fifteen-minute routine my primary care physician (who also happens to be an osteopath) prescribed and printed for me to do every day to help get me out of pain, especially if I was short on time.

Let's begin. We're going to start by doing dynamic warm-up exercises.

A thorough warm-up is one of the most crucial parts in maintaining a healthy back, not to mention healthy muscles and joints throughout the rest of your body. All it takes is five minutes to give your spine a proper warm-up, preparing it for the back strengthening and stretching routines ahead.

Warm-Up

1. Leg Swings (Front to Back)

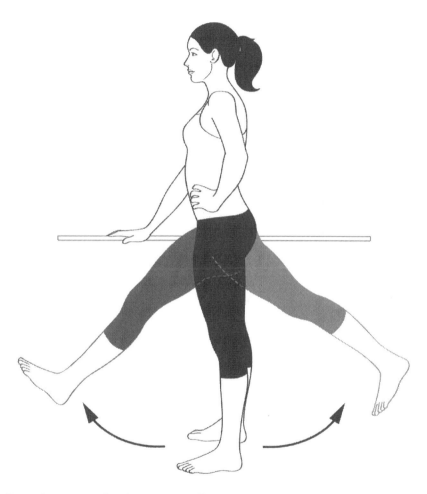

Stand perpendicular to a wall and hold on for support.
Flexing your left foot, swing your left leg forward and back.
Do 10 repetitions with your left leg, and then 10 repetitions
with your right leg.

2. Leg Swings (Side to Side)

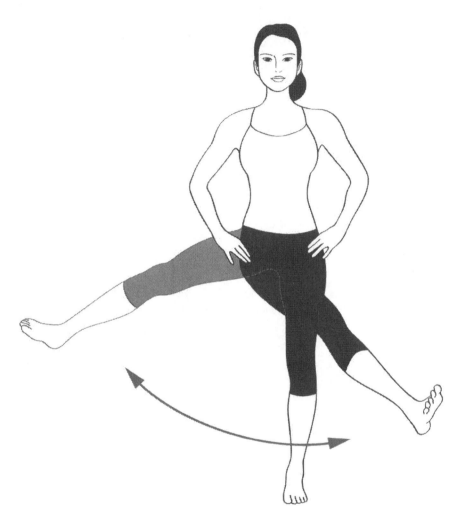

Hold on to your hips, or hold on to the wall at shoulder level and lean into it for support. Swing your left leg to the left, and then across the body to the right. Repeat 10 times with each leg.

3. Ankle Twirls

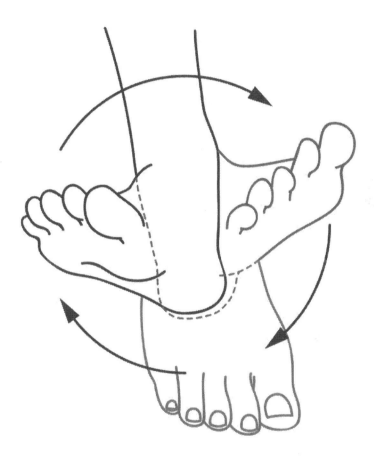

Twirl each ankle 10 times in both directions.

4. Standing Back Extension

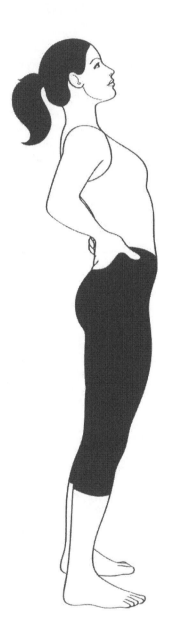

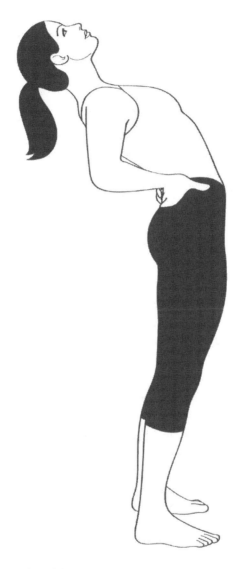

Stand with feet shoulder-width apart. Stretch backward slowly as far as possible, while exhaling for 3 seconds, without bending your knees. Repeat 10 times.

5. Trunk Rotation

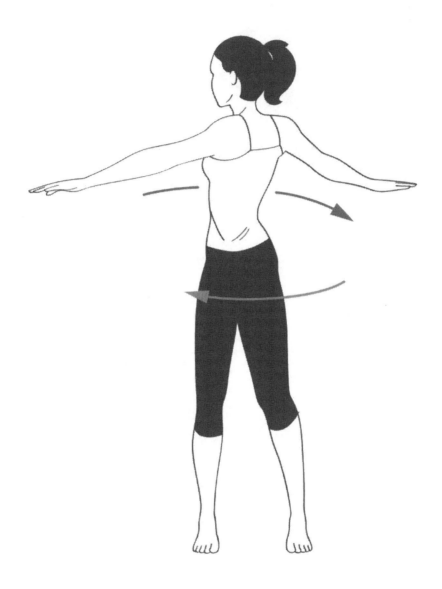

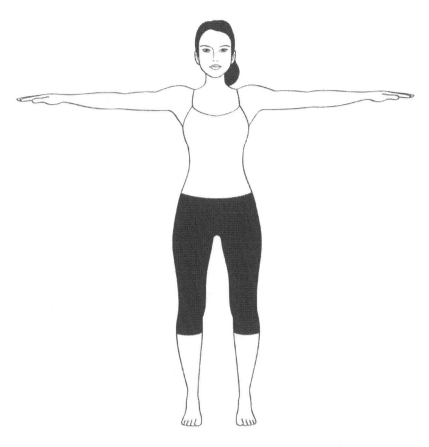

Rotate your body slowly to the right and the left 10 times.

6. Arm Twirls

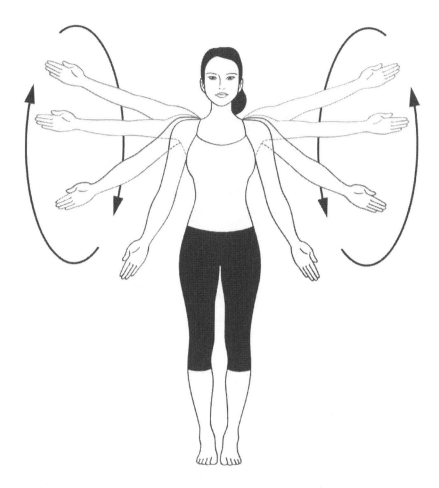

Twirl your arms in circles 10 times forward, and then 10 times backwards.

Let's move on to the next routines, now that you're warmed up.

Getting Started

1. The Plank

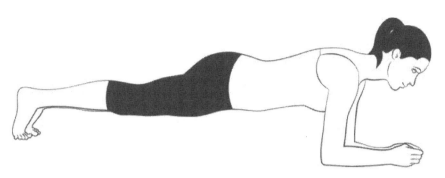

Get into a plank position on the floor with feet hip-width apart and elbows directly under your shoulders.

Brace your core by contracting your abs and attempt to bring your belly button toward your spine.

Keep your back straight and legs and glutes engaged the entire time. Hold this pose for 1 minute.

If 15–30 seconds is all you can do, that's fine, just stay at it. The plank exercise works the transverse abdominus, and this helps you sit up straight, hold your shoulders back, and prevent forward head posture.

You might feel sore, but stay at it. In time you'll be able to work your way up to 1 minute.

Advanced Version Plank with Alternating Arm Raise

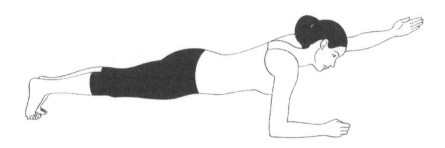

While in the plank position, engage your abs and extend your left arm in front of you. Hold for 2 seconds and then alternate arms. Repeat 10–15 times each side.

The rocking movement of your body as you change arms shifts the load to your core muscles, which in turn have to work harder to maintain your balance.

Tip: Keep your head up, eyes forward, and knees straight.

2. The Side Plank

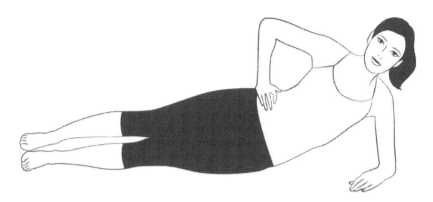

When performing the side plank, start by lying on your side with your forearm on the floor under your shoulder to prop you up, and then stack one foot on top of the other.

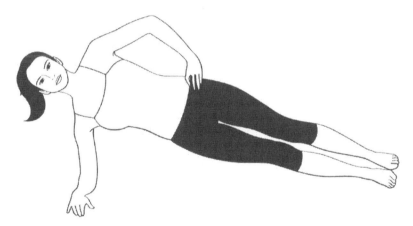

Contract your abdominals and press your forearm into the floor to raise your hips so that your body is straight from your ankles to your shoulders.

Perform six, 10-second holds on each side (do all your holds on one side, and then switch sides). Rest for 20 seconds, then perform four, 10-second holds on each side. Rest for 20 seconds, and then perform three, 10-second holds on each side.

3. Alternating Superman
(or Superwoman) Exercise

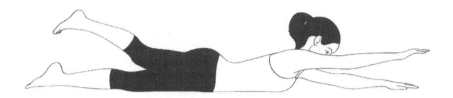

Lie face down on the floor (not a bed) on your stomach with arms and legs extended and your neck in a neutral position.

Lift opposite arm and leg for a count of two, and then repeat 12–15 times. Repeat with the opposite arm and leg.

4. McGill Curl Up

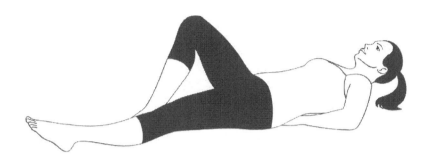

It looks like a crunch, but it's not. Put your hand underneath your lower back to keep your lumbar spine in a slightly neutral position.

Then curl up and focus on the tension in your abdominals.

Perform ten, 5–10 second holds on each side. Do all your holds on one side, and then switch sides.

Now Stretch

When back pain occurs, sometimes it's difficult to stretch the exact spot of pain, because it might be too tender.

A workaround is to stretch the surrounding muscles that are part of the superficial backline, which consists of a line of fascia that starts at the bottom of the foot and travels up the entire posterior (back) side of the body, moving over the head and finishing at the brow bone.

Stretching and lengthening the calves and ankles will help to decrease the stress and tension in the back.

1. Gastrocnemius and Soleus Stretch

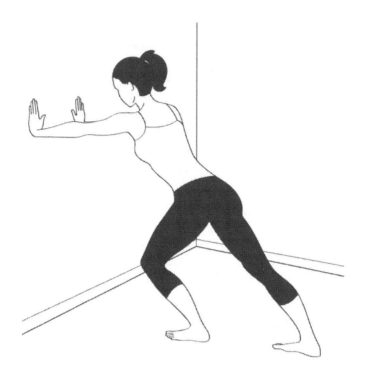

Stand with your legs shoulder-width apart, about 2–3 feet from a wall. When standing, your hands should be able to reach the wall in front of you.

Extend your arms, and place your palms on the wall in front of you.

Lean against the wall and take one step forward with one foot, firmly planting your foot on the floor and bending your leg at the knee.

Make sure the heel of your back foot is firmly planted and your toes are pointing toward the wall. Hold the position for 20–30 seconds and then switch legs.

2. Soleus Stretch

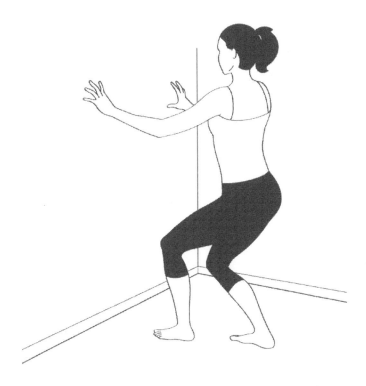

Stand facing a wall and place your hands flat on the wall at about chest height.

Place one leg slightly behind the other, with both your knees bent slightly.

Gently lean toward the wall until you begin to feel the calf stretch. Your heel should remain on the floor during the stretch and should not be elevated.

Stop leaning at the point at which you begin to feel the stretch, then hold the position for 30 seconds. Repeat three times and then switch legs.

3. Standing Hamstring Stretch

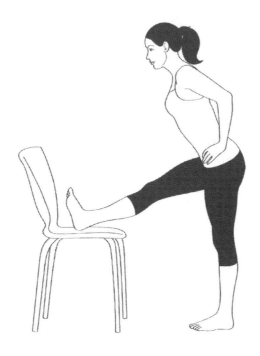

Put your right foot on a support, such as a chair, a table, or a bench. Your foot should be at or below hip level, with your leg straight, your knee and toes pointing straight up, and your quadriceps engaged.

Make sure the hip of your raised leg is not lifted, but rather is releasing downward (without the leg or foot turning outward). Hold for several breaths, repeating on each side.

For a deeper stretch, bend forward over your leg at the hip crease, with your spine and leg straight and your quadriceps firm.

Hold for 30 seconds and switch legs.

4. Hip Flexor Stretch

Did you know that a tight psoas could be causing your back pain?

The psoas muscle is a major hip flexor, located deep in the abdominal contents and spans from the upper portion of the femur to the lumbar vertebrae. It affects your posture and helps to stabilize your spine.

The psoas enables you to walk and run. Every time you lift your knee, it contracts. When your leg swings back, the psoas lengthens.

The psoas often gets short from too much sitting. If your psoas is tight and in a contracted state, it will bring your lower back forward, moving you into an anterior tilt: creating a lordotic curve. This pressure can ultimately compress the joints and discs of the lumbar vertebrae and cause degeneration, which will make them more susceptible to injury.

So regularly stretching your psoas can help prevent future injuries from occurring, or it can mend a chronically tight psoas.

To effectively stretch the hip flexors, first kneel on your right knee, with toes down, and place your left foot flat on the floor in front of you.

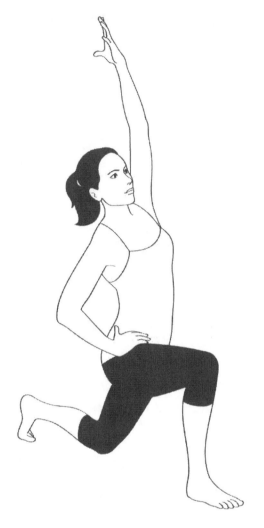

Place your right hand on your left thigh and press your hips forward until you feel a good stretch in the hip flexors. Stretch your non-dominant side first.

Reach your left arm over your head and arch your body back.

Contract your abdominals and slightly tilt your pelvis back, while keeping your chin parallel to the floor. Hold this pose for 30 seconds, and then switch sides.

5. Sideways Lunge Adductor Stretch

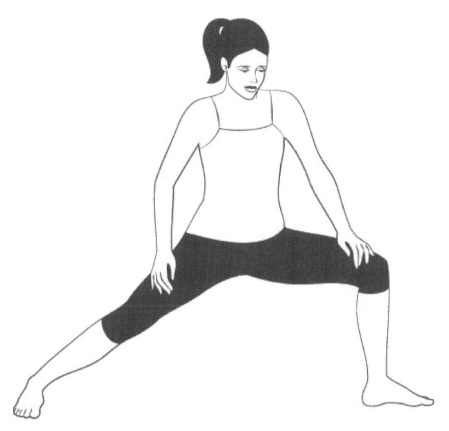

To perform the sideways lunge, keep the rear foot sideways and flat on the floor, and gently bend the front leg, until you feel a gentle stretch along the inside of your leg.

Keep your body upright—there is no need to lean forward. Hold this stretch for 30 seconds, and then repeat with your other leg.

6. Piriformis Stretch (Sitting)

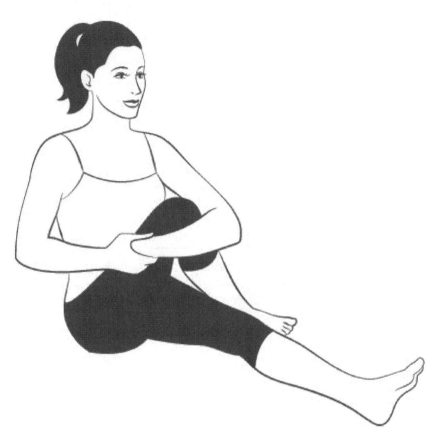

While in a sitting position, cross your right leg over your straightened left leg. Hug your right knee with your left arm, making sure to keep your back straight.

Hold this stretch for 30–60 seconds, and then repeat on the opposite side.

7. Knees to Chest Stretch

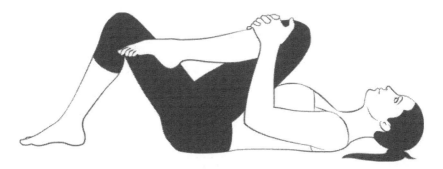

While you're still on your back, with your knees bent, grasp your left knee and pull it to your chest. Hold for 20 seconds.

With your abdominals contracted, try to straighten your right leg. If you experience any discomfort in your back, leave your right leg bent. Repeat this move with the other leg.

Seven Resistance Band Exercises for Low Back Pain

The sedentary lifestyle of desk jockeys (a person who sits in front of a computer all day) makes it difficult to actively use their back muscles. This inevitably leads to slumped back postures and back pain.

Most exercises are body weight or weighted push-pull exercises. These exercises focus on the large, external muscles and are easy to engage physically. When properly utilizing the resistance bands, users have the ability to target the much deeper muscles.

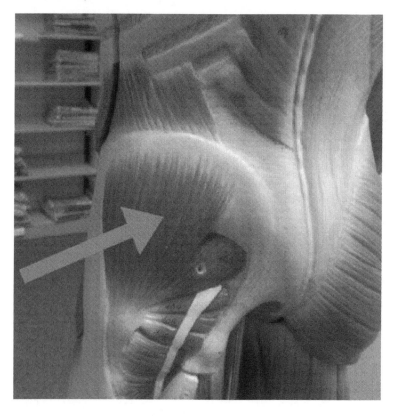

Hip abductor weakness has been implicated as a factor in chronic low back pain. A painful or weak gluteus medius muscle (see blue arrow), the muscle in the buttocks that allows you to laterally rotate the hip, will force a person to lean toward the involved side to place the center of gravity over the hip. This can ultimately lead to abnormal loading of the lumbar spine and subsequent low back pain.

The following seven resistance band exercises will help to stabilize and strengthen the muscles around your hip, which should prove very useful in soothing lower back pain.

What You'll Need

1. Resistance loops http://amzn.to/2oRyHtW

2. Long resistance bands http://amzn.to/2oNbj2a

Recommended Frequency

Do two to three sets of the following seven resistance band exercises for lower back pain three times per week.

1a. Resisted Hip Abduction (Standing)

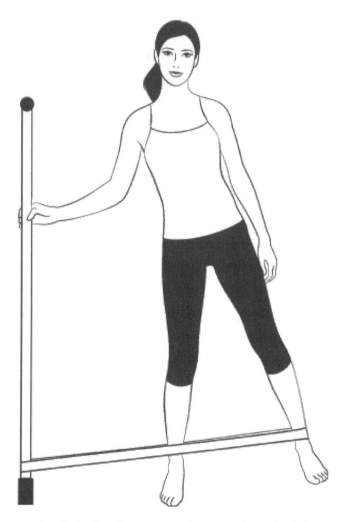

You can substitute the longer resistance band with a resistance band loop.

Do 15–20 repetitions on each side.

Thera-Band hip abductions strengthen the outside of the hip muscles, which help externally rotate and lift your legs to the side.

1b. "The Clam Shell"—Resisted Hip Abduction (Lying Down)

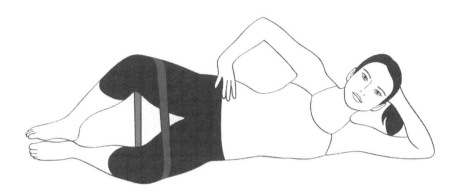

Clam Shells really strengthen hip abductors, because you are lifting them against gravity.

Lying down on your side, with your knees pointed forward and bent at a 90 degree angle, place the resistance band around your knees.

Lift your top knee upwards about 8–2 inches, making sure your top foot stays in place against your bottom foot.

Lower your knee back down to the bottom knee. This completes one repetition. Repeat 15–20 times and then switch sides.

2a. Resisted Hip Extension (Standing)

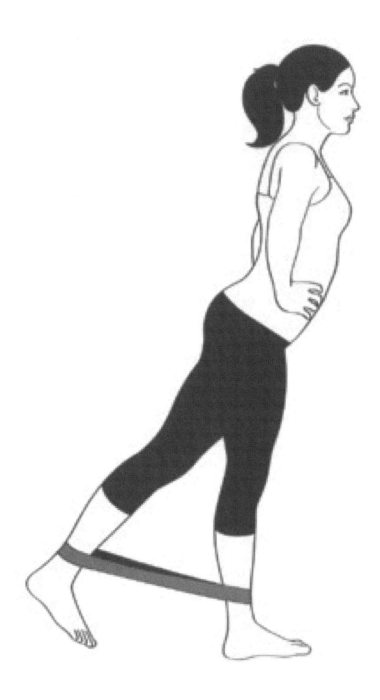

This hip extension exercise strengthens the large buttock muscles, and also the hamstrings on the back of the thigh.

Stand with the band around one ankle and attached to a fixed point in front. Use something to hold onto (like a wall), if you need to.

Keeping the leg straight, extend the hip as far as comfortable and return to the start position.

Keep the hips facing forward and perform the exercise in a slow and controlled manner. You should feel it working the buttock muscles.

Repeat 15–20 times and switch to the other leg, and then do another 15–20 repetitions.

2b. Resisted Hip Extension (Lying Down)

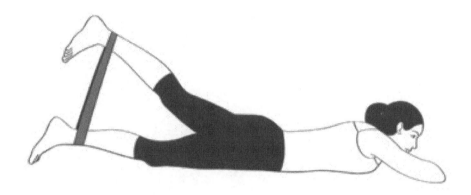

Keep your knee straight and initiate the movement from your hamstrings and glutes

Complete 15–20 repetitions, and then switch to the other leg and do another 15–20 repetitions.

3a. Hamstring Curl with Loop (Standing)

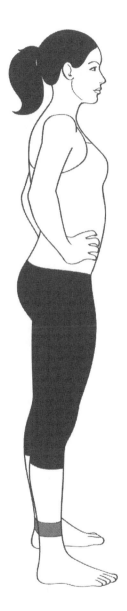

Step into the loop band and stabilize one end of the band around the ankle of the exercising leg and the other end around the left shin.

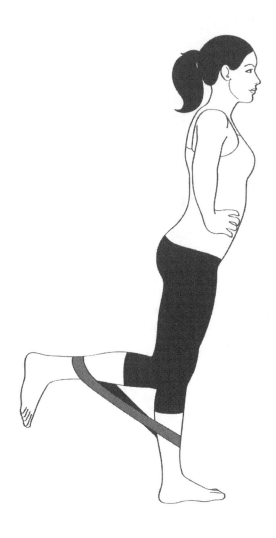

Take a deep breath and exhale as you bend your right knee, curling it up toward your buttocks. Be sure to keep your back straight, your abdominal muscles (abs) engaged, and your eyes fixed on a focal point to help maintain balance. Hold for one breath and slowly return to the starting position.

Complete 15–20 repetitions and then switch to the other leg. Do another 15–20 repetitions.

3b. Hamstring Curl (Seated)

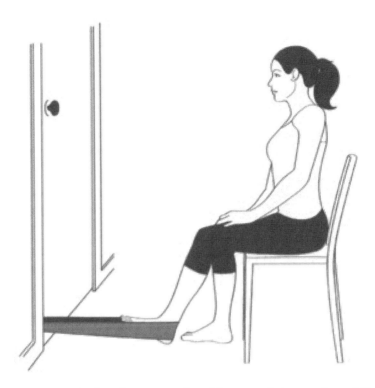

Sitting on a chair, place one heel in a resistance band that is anchored to a door.

In a seated position, place the resistance at the back of the ankle. Begin with the exercising leg pointing straight out, with the knee unlocked.

Begin to bend the knee until it reaches 90 degrees. Then return to the start position. To isolate the hamstrings better, have the toes of the exercising leg pointing toward the face as the exercise is being performed.

Complete 15–20 repetitions and then switch to the other leg. Do another 15–20 repetitions.

4. Straight Leg Dead Lift
(Glute Max and Hamstrings)

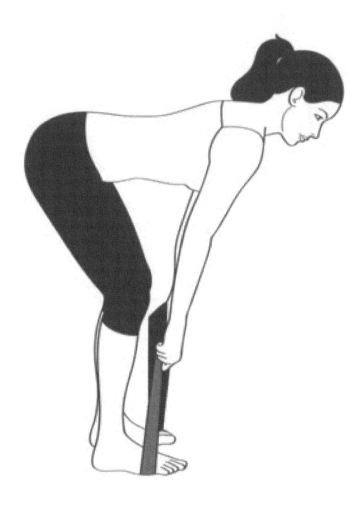

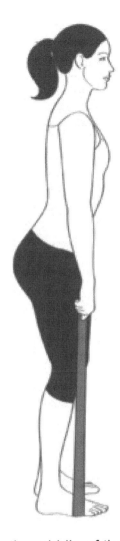

Stand with both feet in the middle of the resistance band. Squat down, and grasp the ends of band in your hands and take up all the slack.

Keep your elbows and back straight and extend your hips and slowly rise from the squat to an upright position.

Repeat 8–12 times. Do three sets.

5. Donkey Kicks

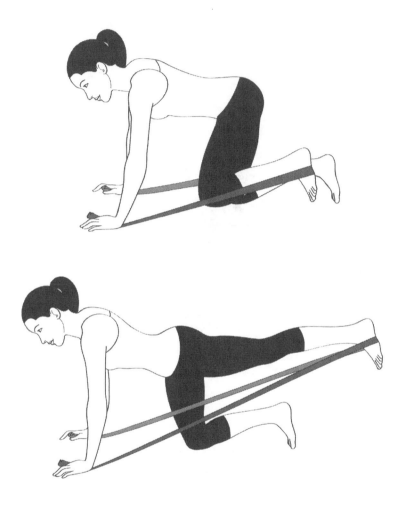

Get down in the all-fours position. Hold the tails of the band with your hands and loop the center around your foot. Kick your leg straight back, while raising your foot slightly toward the ceiling against the resistance of the band. Hold for 1 second at the top, and slowly lower to starting position. Do 15–20 repetitions on each leg.

6. Lateral Squat Walks with Resistance Band

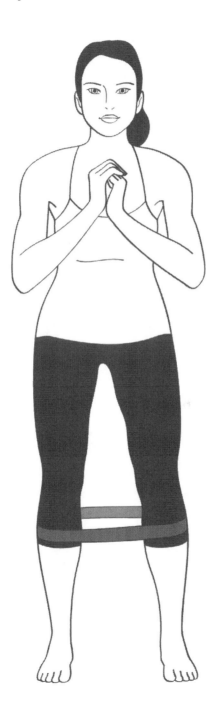

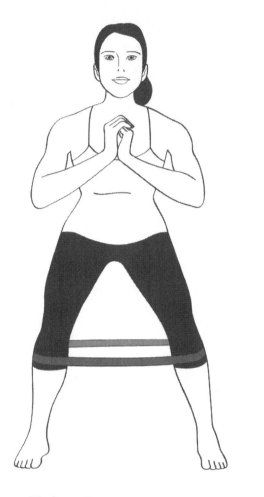

Begin standing with feet directly underneath your hips, abs, and glutes engaged, and hands on your hips.

Squat halfway down and sidestep to the right as far as you can manage without bringing the knees inward.

Bring the left leg toward the right with enough space to keep some resistance in the band. Make sure to look forward and keep your back straight with your toes facing forward.

Step to the right 10 times, then reverse, stepping to the left 10 times. Do three sets.

7. Bridge with Resistance Band

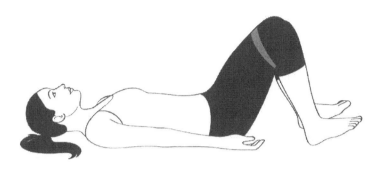

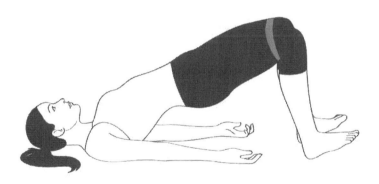

Loop the band tightly around your knees. Separate your knees against the resistance from the band and perform a bridge by lifting your buttocks up off the floor. Slowly return to start position.

Do 15–20 repetitions. Repeat the whole series three times total for an amazingly strong lower body!

Six Foam Rolling Moves to Conquer Back Pain

Myofascial foam rolling can help break down adhesions and scar tissue in the soft tissues of the muscles. Using the weight of your own body, a cylindrical foam roller (purchase this at a fitness center, athletic store, department store, or online) can provide a myofascial release self-massage, smoothing the trigger points, while increasing blood flow and circulation to the soft tissues.

Researchers at Memorial University in Canada published a paper in the January 2014 edition of *Medicine & Science in Sports & Exercise* on the effects of foam rolling as a recovery tool after intense physical activity. The researchers found that foam rolling was beneficial at improving range of motion and reducing delayed onset muscle soreness felt immediately after a hard workout.

When using a foam roller, search for tender areas or trigger points and roll onto these areas, controlling the intensity with your own body weight. Depending on the muscle that you're targeting, you might have to position the roller in a parallel or perpendicular direction, or at a 45-degree angle.

When you find a tender spot, hold sustained pressure on it for a minimum of 20–90 seconds until it "releases." For this to be effective, an individual must be able to relax and breathe while the roller is on a tender spot.

When Is the Best Time to Foam Roll?

After a workout. "Foam rolling 'turns on' your parasympathetic nervous system which is responsible for helping you unwind and recover," says Dr. Kelly Starrett, physical therapist and author of *Becoming a Supple Leopard*.

1. Low Back

With the foam roller resting underneath your low back, pull your right leg up and hug your right knee for 20 seconds. Then roll from the base of your left side of your rib cage to above your glutes.

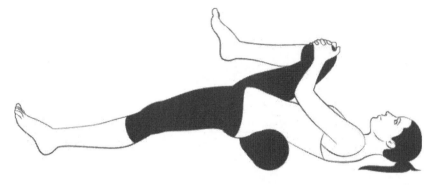

Do 10–12 slow and steady passes, and then repeat on the other side.

2. Glutes

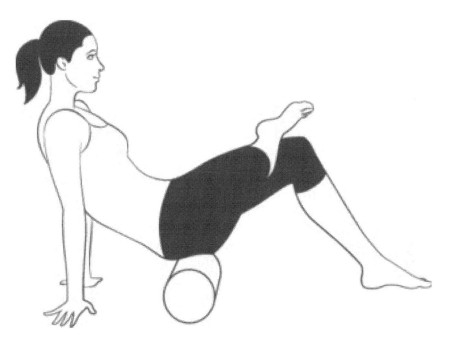

With the foam roller resting underneath both your glutes, bring your right leg up and rest your right ankle above your left knee. Roll onto the side of your right hip. Do 10–12 slow and steady passes. Repeat on the other side.

3. Hamstrings

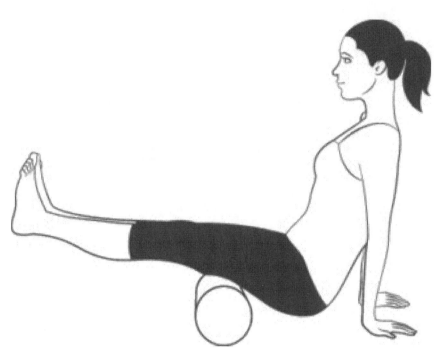

Place the foam roller underneath your upper hamstring muscles below your glutes. Cross your right leg over your left leg and roll the foam roller from your glutes down to right above your left knee. Do 10–12 slow and steady passes. Repeat on the other side.

See https://www.youtube.com/watch?v=fMfe6DnlGvA

4. Quadriceps and Hip Flexors

Because your hip flexors are located slightly toward the outer portion of your pelvic region, it's more effective to roll with just one thigh rather than on both sides at the same time.

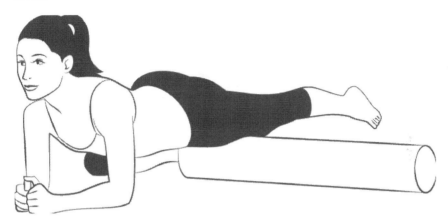

Start face down on the floor in a plank position with one thigh on the foam roller. As you roll up and down on your hip flexors, slightly rotate right to left to seek and destroy any knots or trigger points. Continue until you hit the entire front side of your thigh. Do 10–12 slow and steady passes up and down the quad. Repeat on the other side.

5. Foam Roll along Length of Back

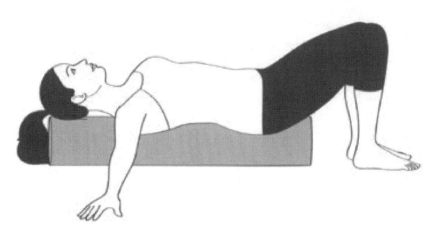

Place the foam roller vertically. Lay down on it with your head at one end and backside at the other end.

Let your arms relax to side with your palms up or down.

Lie there for up to 15 minutes.

6. Foam Roll Spinal Release

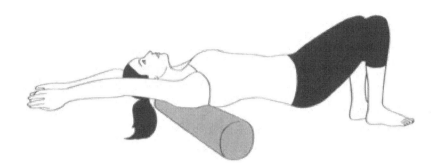

With this foam roller stretch, you won't be rolling at all; you'll be using your arms for the movement. Place your arms down at your sides. Keeping them completely straight, lift them up and over your head until they are touching the floor behind you (like you're raising your arms in excitement). You can also raise them sideways, mimicking a snow angel type of movement.

Tip: make sure you relax your body and completely open your chest, so that you're making the most out of this exercise. The key here is to stretch and relax your muscles; you're not massaging anything with this exercise.

If you find the foam roller too big to roll out the knots in your mid and lower back, try using the time-tested tennis ball method.

Stretching is not enough when it comes to releasing a knotted muscle. If you can't carve out the time to schedule a professional, deep-tissue massage, or you can't fit one into your budget, performing a self-massage with a tennis ball or foam roller can be a cost-effective alternative.

Three Foam Rolling Mistakes When Rolling Away Back Pain

1. Don't Roll Directly Where the Pain Is

A painful area might be the result of tension imbalances elsewhere in your body. Plus, rolling a painful, inflamed area might increase inflammation and inhibit healing. It's often best to roll just a few inches away from a highly sensitive area first, and then use large, sweeping motions to cover the entire area.

2. Avoid Rolling Too Quickly

Your movements on the foam roller should be slow and concentrated. If you roll too fast, your muscles won't have time to adapt to and manage the compression, and you're not going to eliminate adhesions.

3. Don't Spend Too Much Time on Knots

It's OK to work on your knots using the foam roller, but if you spend 5–10 minutes on the same spot, you could cause damage to the tissue or nerves. This is especially true if you also attempt to place your entire weight on the knot.

Ideally, you should spend just 20 seconds, or so, on each tender spot, while managing how much pressure you apply. When using a foam roller, you should apply enough pressure so that you feel some tension released, either with constant pressure or by making small movements back and forth. A mild amount of discomfort is expected, but you shouldn't be in pain.

This is counterproductive because rolling your lower back will cause your spinal muscles to contract to protect your spine. To release your lower back, try rolling the muscles that connect to it, including your piriformis (located within your glutes), hip flexors, and rectus femoris (a main muscle in your quads), according to National Academy of Sports Medicine certified personal trainer Monica Vazquez.

The Ninety-Second, Tennis-Ball Method for Low Back Pain Relief

Using a tennis ball (or lacrosse ball) to work out the knots and tight spots in the low back is a time-honored pastime for many self-massage enthusiasts. Tennis balls can easily grip the skin and sink in and loosen up the thoraco-lumbar fascia (that's the connective tissue in the low back).

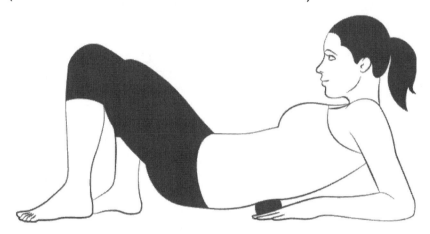

Start by lying on the floor and propping yourself on your elbows. Then lift your bottom and place two tennis balls on either side of your lower spine.

Let your body slowly ease onto the two balls, and then use your arms to help you glide down toward your heels and then back up, just below your ribcage, and then back down again. Continue doing this for 90 seconds, or about 8–12 repetitions.

If this position starts to strain your neck and shoulders, rest your head and upper body on the floor and place the balls in the groove on either side of your lower spine. Then rock your hips side to side, like an excited dog slowly wagging its tail. You should feel the tension and tightness in your low back melt away.

Got a Pain in the Butt? Try This!

You can try self trigger-point therapy using a ball. Find a painful spot in the glutes, place the ball at that location, and then relax your body into the ball.

Hold this position for 20 seconds or so on each tender spot or until you notice a significant reduction in pain. Move to the next painful spot. The total time spent on this exercise should be no more than 5–10 minutes.

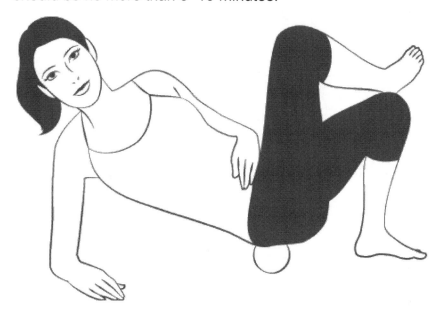

What Can Jelly Donuts Teach You about Bulging and Herniated Discs?

Using the analogy of the jelly donut is an easy way to visualize the more complex anatomy of spinal discs. Simply put, the spinal discs are made up of two main parts—the jelly-like disc center, called the nucleus pulposus, and the outermost layer of collagen rings, called the annulus fibrosis. These two parts help the discs move and protect the vertebrae.

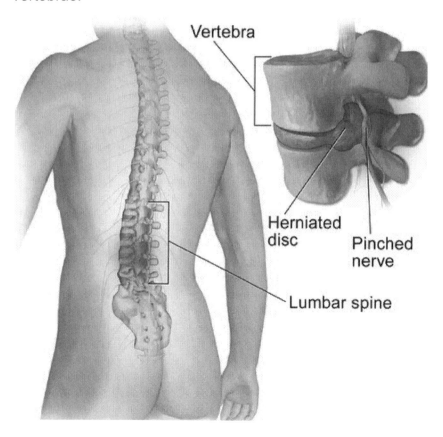

Vertebra

Herniated disc

Pinched nerve

Lumbar spine

When someone has a **bulging disc**, the outer layer of the spinal disc extends outside the vertebral space, resembling a hamburger that's too big for its bun (that's right, another fast-food analogy). Research indicates that more than 50 out of 100 people who had a pain-free back and had a magnetic resonance imaging (MRI) tested positive for a bulging disk. A bulging disc is considered to be a common part of the disc's aging process and usually doesn't cause any pain.

A **slipped or herniated disc** is a whole other ball game. This happens when the tough outer layer of the disc degenerates, or sustains a trauma and cracks, allowing some of the nucleus pulposa to protrude out of the disc into the spinal canal. Herniations are most common in the fourth and fifth lumbar vertebrae. This weak spot lies directly under the spinal nerve root, putting direct pressure on the nerves causing radiating pain, tingling, and numbness down the leg.

These symptoms of a herniated disc are called sciatica or lumber radiculopathy. Some other common symptoms of a disc tear or herniated disc are . . .

- The pain came on suddenly without any injury or physical trauma.

- It's painful to bend over, even just a little bit.

- Sitting hurts, even when done for a few minutes.

- Sneezing and coughing make the pain worse.

What Causes a Disc to Herniate or "Go Out" and How to Fix It

If you're like most people in today's world, you probably sit—at work, in a car, on the couch—for extended periods. Your spine is flexed forward for a large portion of the day. Then, if you go to the gym and perform weight-bearing exercises that round your back, such as deadlifts, squats, kettlebell swings, or shoulder presses, you're setting yourself up for a potential bulging or herniated disc.

Even if you're not a gym rat and only sporadically workout, simply bending to tie your shoes can make your back go out.

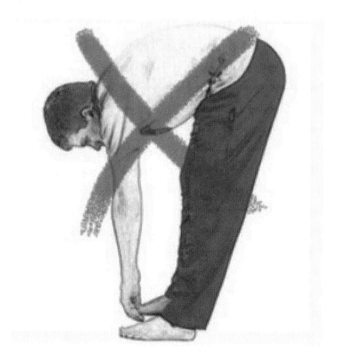

You see, each time you forward bend, your donut or spinal disc gets pinched at the front, and chances are, if it's frequent enough or hard enough, the annulus will break, letting the jelly or nucleus leak out and push onto the nerve. Any pressure on the nerve will instantly lead to inflammation and pain.

So, what's the solution to fixing a herniated disc? You need to push the donut or disc to the opposite side!

The Six-Minute Emergency Back Pain Treatment That's Safe for Herniated and Bulging Discs

The following two exercises can push a herniated lumber disc back into place.

When your back is in an acute phase with a painful back spasm, and it hurts to even tie your shoe, before you do any stretching or strengthening exercises, you want to first decrease the level of pain.

The following exercises are taken from *Treat Your Own Back* by Robin McKenzie, a New Zealand-born physiotherapist whose McKenzie Method is currently the most studied diagnostic treatment system for back pain.

Repeat these two exercises 6–8 times throughout the day until you go to bed.

1. Press Up on Elbows

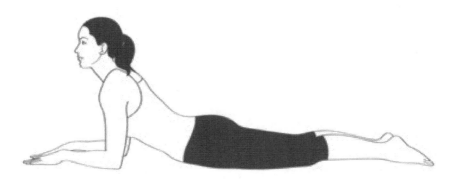

Lie on your stomach on the floor with legs extended and hands palm down just above shoulders. Retract your shoulder blades down and in toward the midline of your spine. Maintaining that position, lift your chest off the floor and extend through the spine from your tailbone to the top of your neck; allow your back to arch.

Remain in this position for 2–3 minutes, keeping the back of your neck long and making sure your front hip bones stay in contact with the floor during the entire movement.

2. Fully Extended Press Up

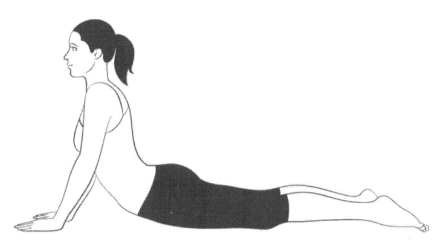

Press your palms into the floor and lift your upper body, keeping hips and pelvis rooted to the floor. Extend through the spine from the tailbone to the neck, allowing your back to arch.

Hold for 2 seconds, and then slowly lower to the start position for one rep. Do 10 reps.

How do you know it's working?

You know it's improving when the pain moves out of the leg and/or hip region and into the center of the low back. Or if the pain's already in the center of your back, it becomes more focused into a small point. This is what Robin McKenzie refers to as "centralization."

If you get the pain to centralize, you're effectively pushing the protruding jelly back inside the spinal disc and safely away from the nearby nerves.

If at any point while you're doing the press up exercise, you feel radiating pain down your leg, then stop.

In this case, you should lie face down on your stomach for 5–10 minutes, and then slowly make an effort to do the press up on elbows and then gradually move into the fully extended press up.

If the pain persists to shoot down the leg, or the sciatic leg pain worsens, contact your doctor.

If you're unable to lie down where you are (say you're at work), then doing a standing back extension will suffice.

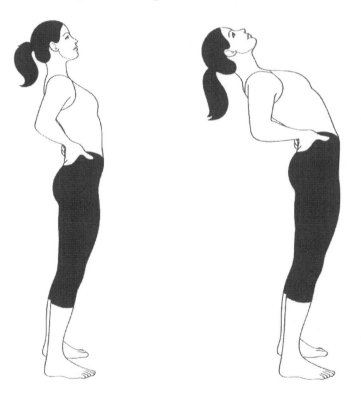

Stand with feet shoulder-width apart. Stretch backwards slowly as far as possible, while exhaling for 3 seconds, without bending your knees. Repeat 10 times.

Tip: Do these every 20–30 minutes and refer to the **Sit the Right Way** section of this book for good sitting posture.

This One Simple Move Can Melt a Back Spasm in Just Five Minutes

Sometimes that pain in your lower back has nothing to do with your lower back. Instead, a problem is located somewhere else, such as a shoulder misalignment, uneven hips, or a tilted pelvis is really the culprit. When you correct these other imbalances, the back pain eases. That's the thinking behind the Egoscue Method, a nonmedical technique that incorporates stretches and exercises that realign the body and restore proper muscle and joint function. The technique is based on the concept that pain occurs when biomechanical imbalances place abnormal stress on muscles and ligaments.

When back pain is extreme, in the case of a herniated disk, many people assume the answer is surgery. But medical intervention comes with risks, a long recovery process, and, often, more pain. Another way to correct and avoid musculoskeletal lower back pain is through corrective daily movements, such as the Static Back position recommended by Egoscue.

The Static Back

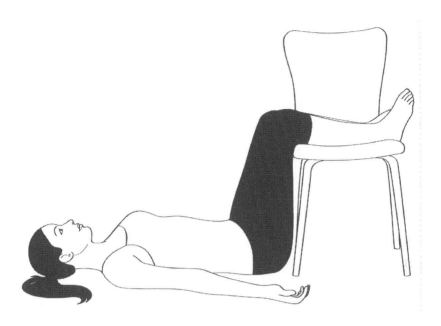

Lie on the floor with your legs resting on a chair. Rest your arms at your side at a 45-degree angle with palms up.

Take deep breaths and let your upper body relax and the curve of your lower back flatten to the floor. Hold this position for 5 minutes.

Top Seven Exercises to Prevent Future Back Spasms and Herniated Discs

The following exercise routine is easy on the spinal discs, while building core stability for maximum protection, so that you can prevent future flare-ups. It targets the front, back, and sides of your core, while removing gravity and supporting your spine at both ends.

Repeat these exercises 3–4 per times per week.

1. Press Ups

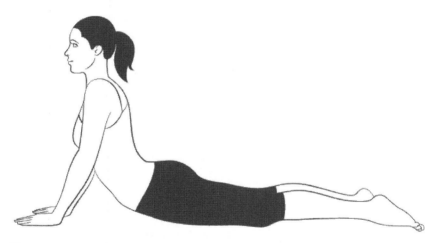

Press your palms into the floor and lift your upper body, keeping hips and pelvis rooted to the floor. Extend through the spine from the tailbone to the neck, allowing your back to arch.

Hold for 2 seconds, and then slowly lower back to the start position for one rep. Do 10 reps.

2. Cat/Cow Pose

Starting on your hands and knees, an all-fours position, move into the Cat Pose by slowly pressing your spine up, arching your back.

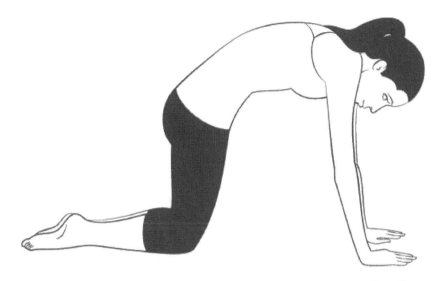

Hold the pose for a few seconds, and then move to the Cow Pose by scooping your spine in, pressing your shoulder blades back, and lifting your head.

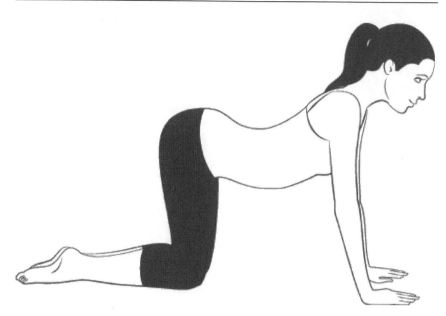

Moving back and forth from Cat Pose to Cow Pose helps move your spine to a neutral position, relaxing the muscles and easing tension.

Repeat the sequence 10 times, flowing smoothly from cat to cow, and cow back to cat.

3. Bird Dog Pose (Kneeling Superman/Superwoman)

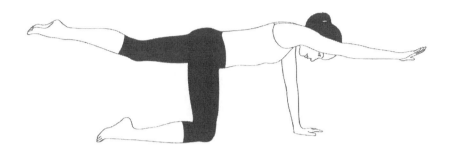

Start with the all-fours position, tighten your hamstrings, glutes, and low back and lift to straighten your leg and opposite arm while maintaining proper alignment. Make sure to push through your heel.

Perform six, 10-second holds on each side (do all your holds on one side, and then switch sides). Rest for 20 seconds, and then perform four, 10-second holds on each side. Rest for 20 seconds, and then perform three, 10-second holds on each side.

4. The Side Plank

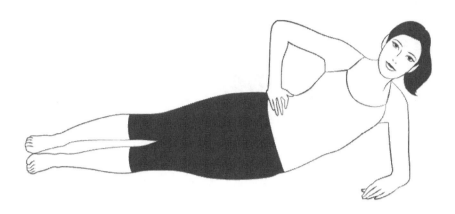

When performing the side plank, start by lying on your side with your forearm on the floor under your shoulder, to prop you up, and then stack your feet on top of each other.

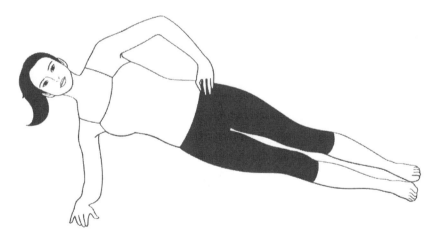

Contract your abdominals and press your forearm into the floor to raise your hips, so that your body is straight from your ankles to your shoulders.

Perform six, 10-second holds on each side (do all your holds on one side, and then switch sides). Rest for 20 seconds, and then perform four, 10-second holds on each side. Rest for 20 seconds, and then perform three, 10-second holds on each side.

5. McGill Curl Up

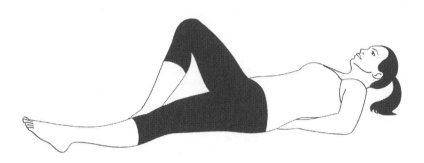

It looks like a crunch, but it's not. Put your hand underneath your lower back to keep your lumbar spine in a slightly neutral position.

Then curl up and focus on the tension in your abdominals.

Perform six, 10-second holds on each side (do all your holds on one side, and then switch sides). Rest for 20 seconds, and then perform four, 10-second holds on each side. Rest for 20 seconds, and then perform three, 10-second holds on each side.

6a. Bridge Exercise

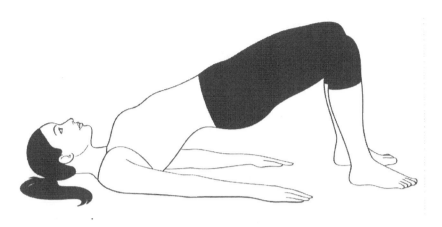

Lie on your back with your hips and knees bent to 90 degrees, with your feet flat on the floor and arms palm down by your sides. Take a deep breath in and, as you breathe out, lift your hips off the floor until shoulders, hips, and knees are in a straight line.

Hold about 6 seconds, and then slowly lower hips to the floor. Repeat 8–12 times.

6b. Advanced Bridge with Knee Pillow Squeeze

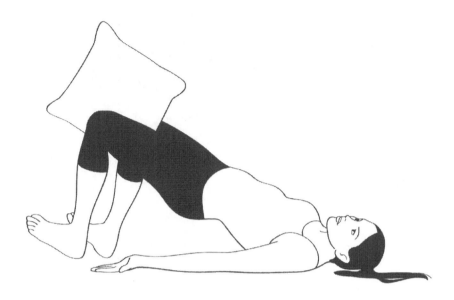

This exercise helps to rebalance the pelvis. Start in the bridge position and place a pillow between your inner thighs. Tuck in your tailbone and tense your abs, as you lift your hips, pushing down equally on both feet.

Squeezing the pillow tight, hold in top position for 1 minute.

7. Straight Leg Dead Lift
(Glut Max and Hamstrings)

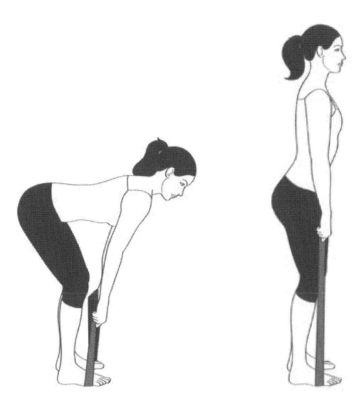

Stand in middle of the resistance band with both feet. Squat and grasp the ends of the band in your hands and take up all slack. Keep your elbows and back straight and extend your hips. Slowly return from the squat to an upright position.

Repeat 8–12 times. Do three sets.

Do these seven exercises and you'll actually *feel* tighter and stronger in your core and this will help prevent a future back flareup.

Sleep This Way: Worst Sleep Positions for Back Pain

Experts believe that people with sleep problems experience more problems with back pain. "Sleep deprivation is known to affect mood and functional ability and negatively impacts perception of pain," says Dr. Santhosh Thomas, a spine specialist with the Cleveland Clinic.

According to the National Sleep Foundation, when you're in pain, it negatively affects your quality of sleep, resulting in a lighter sleep state and more frequent waking throughout the night.

A good night's sleep can help improve the severity of pain, overall mood, and the ability to function, according to a study published in the November 2016 issue of the *Annals of Behavioral Medicine*.

Worst Sleep Position for Back Pain

Some sleep positions can lead to painful cricks and place unnecessary pressure on your neck, shoulders, hips, lower back, knees, and even your heels. Finding the perfect sleep position that is immune to back pain is like finding a four-leaf clover, but there are a few positions you can master that can help you achieve more restful sleep.

What's the Worst Position for Back Pain?

Sleeping on your stomach. Generally, sleeping on your stomach can flatten the natural curve of your spine, putting added strain on your back muscles and lead to a crick in the neck because of the awkward, rotated head position. Also, avoid using a pillow for your head, if it places your neck or back in a strained position

Forget about trying to maintain the same position all night. It's completely normal for you to wiggle around and shift your body while you're trying to catch some shut-eye. In fact, it's a good thing, because a little movement can help reduce the pressure on your back. However, on the flip side, if you stay in a position for too long, it can intensify back pain.

The Best Way to Sleep, If You Have Back Pain

A 2011 study evaluating pain and sleep, published in *European Spine Journal*, found that 58.7 percent of people suffering with low back pain experienced sleep disturbances. I've had countless clients who come to me saying that they woke up feeling stiff and achy, probably from "sleeping wrong."

See http://www.everydayhealth.com/news/switch-sleep-positions-ease-back-pain/

What IS the Right Way to Sleep If You Have Low Back Pain?

By making simple changes in your sleeping position, you can take strain off your back. If you sleep on your side, draw your legs up slightly toward your chest and put a pillow between your legs. Use a full-length body pillow if you prefer.

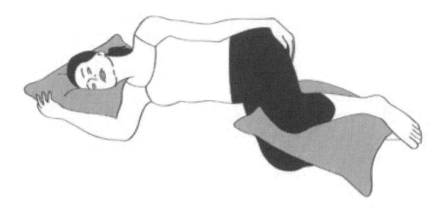

Lying on your side with a pillow between your knees will help to reduce any curve in your spine and ease the pressure on your spinal discs.

Try to keep your top leg from falling over your bottom leg. You also can put a small, rolled-up towel under your waist.

If you sleep on your back, place a pillow under your knees to help maintain the normal curve of your lower back. You might try a small, rolled towel under the small of your back for additional support. Support your neck with a pillow.

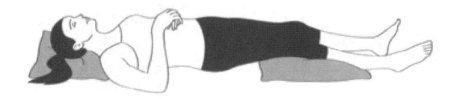

Check Your Bed

According to a 2010 study in *Applied Ergonomics*, if you have low back pain, getting a medium to firm mattress layered with memory foam might be the best choice for reducing your pain and improving your quality of sleep.

In fact, as stated in the study, 63 percent reported significant improvements in low back pain after switching to a new sleep system. If your current mattress is more than 10 years old, it's probably time to get a new one.

An old, lumpy bed and the position you sleep in can cause your back to become strained during that valuable rest time. This "can actually increase stress on our ligaments, spinal discs and spinal joints," says Dr. Robert Oexman, director of the Sleep to Live Institute.

See http://www.mayoclinic.org/diseases-conditions/back-pain/multimedia/sleeping-positions/sls-20076452

See http://www.wikihow.com/Sleep-With-Lower-Back-Pain

Before You Roll Out of Bed . . .

When your alarm clock rings or buzzes in the morning, do you leap out of bed, as if you've been struck by lightning, or do you hit the snooze button?

Dr. Oexman says your answer should be, "Stretch my back!" He says that the "greatest incidence of slipped discs occurs within 30 to 60 minutes after we wake up."

Oexman recommends that you "stretch out your back before you ever leave bed," instead of falling back to sleep, which interrupts your natural sleep pattern, counteracting sleep's restorative values.

The following four stretches can make a powerful difference in preventing back pain and keeping you limber throughout the day.

First, to rise from bed:

- Roll onto your side and bend both knees.

- Drop your feet over the side of the bed, as you push with both arms to sit up.

- Scoot to the edge of the bed and position your feet under your buttocks.

- Stand up, keeping your back in the neutral position.

See http://www.webmd.com/back-pain/sleeping-positions-for-people-with-low-back-pain

Roll Out of Bed the Right Way

Don't Roll Out of Bed before You Do These Four Moves

1. Low Back Stretch

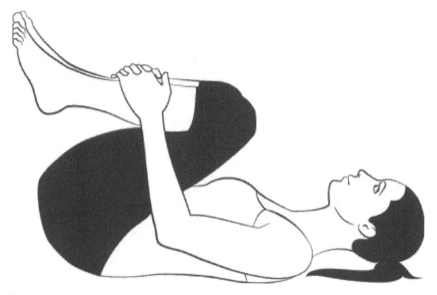

Bring both your knees to your chest. Start by first raising one and then holding the knee with both hands. Then raise the other knee. Grasping both your knees, pull them toward your chest.

Hold this stretch for 30 seconds.

2. Piriformis Stretch

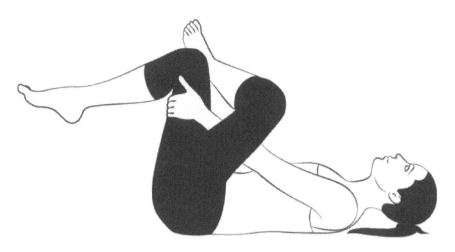

The piriformis muscle runs through the glutes and can contribute to back and leg pain.

Lying on your back with both knees bent, cross your left leg over your right leg. Using both hands, reach under your right knee and pull it toward your chest. You should feel a stretch in the glutes on your left side.

Hold this stretch for 30 seconds and then repeat with your other leg.

3. Pelvic Tilt

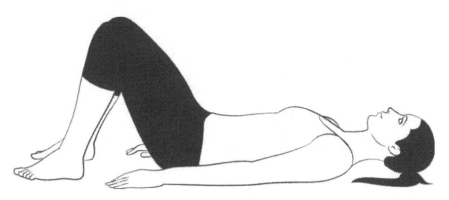

Lie on your back with your knees bent. In this relaxed position, the small of your back will not be touching the floor. Tighten your abdominal muscles, so that the small of your back presses against the bed. Hold this pose for 5 seconds, and then relax. Repeat 10 times.

4. Knees to Chest Stretch

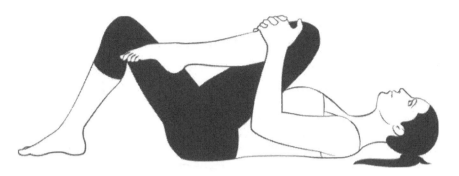

While you're still on your back, with your knees bent, grasp your left knee and pull it to your chest.

With your abdominals contracted, try to straighten your right leg. If you experience any discomfort in your back, leave your right leg bent.

Hold this stretch for 30 seconds and then repeat with your other leg.

Now, you can confidently roll out of bed the right way.

Conclusion

Taking ownership of your pain is essential to living a pain-free life. I hope that the various ways illustrated in this book have empowered you to take action so you can feel like yourself again.

As the old saying goes, "motion is lotion for the joints." What that means is that the older you get, the less lubrication (or synovial fluid) you produce for your joints. And the little fluid you do produce isn't absorbed as well by the joints, so the more active you are, the better you'll feel overall.

Watch some young children, and you'll instantly notice how active they are and how they're naturally inclined to be constantly moving. When recess rolls around, what do they do? Sit on their bums and veg out? Nope! They run around like bolts of lightning and hop, skip, and jump.

This is a learning opportunity for back pain sufferers. Instead of resting the back by doing less, activity is essential to reversing the debilitating effects of back pain.

I wish you well on your journey to health and well-being!

References

Got Back Pain? Now What? Nine Common Back Pain Myths

Bichell, Rae Ellen. (2016). "Forget the Gizmos: Exercise Works Best for Lower-Back Pain." See http://www.npr.org/sections/healthshots/2016/01/11/4623663 61/forget-the-gizmos-exercise-works-best-for-lower-back-pain.

Cole, Andrew J. (2000). "The Myths and Reality of Back Pain and Back Problems." See http://www.spine-health.com/conditions/lower-back-pain/myths-and-reality-back-pain-and-back-problems.

Deardorff, William W. (2017). "Types of Back Pain: Acute Pain, Chronic Pain, and Neuropathic Pain." See http://www.spine-health.com/conditions/chronic-pain/types-back-pain-acute-pain-chronic-pain-and-neuropathic-pain.

"Handout on Health: Back Pain." (2013). National Institutes of Health (NIH): National Institute of Arthritis and Musculoskeletal and Skin Diseases. See http://www.niams.nih.gov/Health_Info/Back_Pain/default.asp.

Hoy, D., Bain, C., Williams, G., March, L., Brooks, P., Blyth, F. Woolf, A., Vos, T., Buchbinder, R. (2012). "A Systemic Review of the Global Prevalence of Low Back Pain." *Arthritis & Rheumatology* 64, no. 6, 2028–2037. doi: 10.1002/art.34347.

Institute of Medicine of the National Academies (2011). *Relieving Pain in America, A Blueprint for Transforming Prevention, Care, Education, and Research.* Washington, DC: The National Academies Press.

"Low Back Pain Fact Sheet." (2003). National Institutes of Health (NIH): National Institute of Neurological Disorders and Stroke. See http://www.ninds.nih.gov/disorders/backpain/detail_backpain.htm.

"Low Back Pain Fact Sheet." (2014). National Institute of Neurological Disorders and Stroke. See http://www.ninds.nih.gov/disorders/backpain/detail_backpain.htm.

Malmivaara, A., Häkkinen, U., Aro, T., Heinrichs, M-L., Koskenniemi, L., Kuosma, E., Lappi, S., Paloheimo, R., Servo, C., Vaaranen, V., and Hernberg, S., (1995). "The Treatment of Acute Low Back Pain—Bed Rest, Exercises, or Ordinary Activity?" *The New England Journal of Medicine* 332, 351–355.

Steffens, D., Maher, C.G., Pereira, L.S.M. (2016). "Prevention of Low Back Pain: A Systematic Review and Meta-analysis." *JAMA Intern Med* 176, no. 2,199–208. doi: 10.1001/jamainternmed.2015.7431

Four Most Common Causes of Back Pain

McKenzie, Robin A. (2011). Treat Your Own Back. Orthopedic Physical Therapy Products.

Sit the Right Way

"Low Back Pain Fact Sheet." (2003). National Institutes of Health (NIH): National Institute of Neurological Disorders and Stroke. See http://www.ninds.nih.gov/disorders/backpain/detail_backpain.htm.

Two Accessories

Coccyx Orthopedic Memory Foam Seat Cushion

http://amzn.to/2pkQx8f

McKenzie Lumbar Roll

http://amzn.to/2nNDnU5

Get Up, Stand Up

Alexandre, Misato. (2015). "9 Worst Exercises for Your Back." See http://www.fitwirr.com/fitness/-worst-exercises-lower-back.

Iliades, Chris. (2014). "The Best and Worst Exercises for Back Pain." See http://www.everydayhealth.com/back-pain-pictures/the-best-and-worst-exercises-for-back-pain.aspx#04.

"Low Back Pain: What Can You Do?" (2016). See http://www.webmd.com/back-pain/lower-back-pain-10/slideshow-exercises.

Munoz, Kissairis. (2013). "The 10 Worst Exercises to Do If You Have Back Pain." See http://www.rodalewellness.com/fitness/back-pain-exercises/slide/2.

"Preventing Back Pain at Work and at Home." (2012). American Academy of Orthopaedic Surgeons. See http://orthoinfo.aaos.org/topic.cfm?topic=A00175.

"Walking Could Help Ease Lower Back Pain, Study Finds." (2013). See http://www.huffingtonpost.com/2013/03/12/back-pain-walking_n_2838560.html.

Twenty-One Day, Low Back Pain, Relief Program

"Lumbar/Core Strength and Stability Exercises." See https://uhs.princeton.edu/sites/uhs/files/documents/Lumbar.pdf.

Ten Stretches and Eleven Core and Back-Strengthening Exercises

"Adductor Assisted Back Extension." (2014). See https://www.youtube.com/watch?v=mZr5ywYLSwQ.

"Advanced Workout: Plank with Arm Lift." (2009). See http://www.womenshealthmag.com/fitness/advanced-workout-plank-with-arm-lift.

Ameel. (2012). "Weak Posterior Kinetic Chain: Cause of Lower Back Pain." See http://backpainsolutionsonline.com/announcements-and-releases/backpain/lower-back-pain-causes/weak-posterior-kinetic-chain-cause-of-lower-back-pain.

Ferris, Tim. (2010). The Four-Hour Body: An Uncommon Guide to Rapid Fat-Loss, Incredible Sex, and Becoming Superhuman. Harmony, 352.

Goodman, Eric. (2011). *Foundation: Redefine Your Core, Conquer Back Pain, and Move with Confidence*. Rodale Books, 96–97.

"Hamstring Stretches." See http://www.stretching-exercises-guide.com/hamstring-stretches.html.

Koch, Nathan. (2014). "New Runner: Dynamic Stretching vs. Static Stretching." See http://running.competitor.com/2014/07/injury-prevention/dynamic-stretching-vs-static-stretching_54248#uHp6YUjcUOp00fxy.99.

Samartzis, D., Karppinen, J., Chan, D., Luk, K.D.K., and Cheung, K.M.C. (2012). "The Association of Lumbar Intervertebral Disc Degeneration on Magnetic Resonance Imaging with Body Mass Index in Overweight and Obese Adults: A Population-Based Study." *Arthritis & Rheumatology* 64, no. 5, 1488–1496. doi: 10.1002/art.33462.

Shiri, R., Karppinen, J., Leino-Arjas, P., Solovieva, S., and Viikari-Juntura, E. (2010). "The Association between Obesity and Low Back Pain: A Meta-Analysis." *American Journal of Epidemiology* 171, no. 2, 135–154. doi: 10.1093/aje/kwp356.

Shiri, R., Solovieva, S., Husgafvel-Pursiainen, K., Taimela, S., Saarikoski, L.A., Huupponen, R., Viikari, J., Raitakari, O.T., and Viikari-Juntura, E. (2008). "The Association between Obesity and the Prevalence of Low Back Pain in Young Adults: The Cardiovascular Risk in Young Finns

Study." *American Journal of Epidemiology* 167, no. 9, 1110–1119. doi: 10.1093/aje/kwn007.

Westbrock, H. (2015). "The Best Stretch for Your Hip Flexors—The 'Couch Stretch.'" See https://premiersportsandspine.com/2015/06/the-best-stretch-for-your-hip-flexors-the-couch-stretch/.

Seven Resistance Band Exercises for Low Back Pain

Bailey, Aubrey. (2011). "The Best Back Exercises with Resistance Bands. See http://www.livestrong.com/article/387924-the-best-back-exercises-with-resistance-bands/

Myosource Kinetic Bands. See https://myosource.com/back-pain/

"Thera-Band Exercises for Lower Back Pain Relief." http://www.anteriorpelvictilthq.com/thera-band-exercises-for-lower-back-pain-relief/

What You'll Need

Long Resistance Bands

> http://amzn.to/2oNbj2a

Resistance Loops

> http://amzn.to/2oRyHtW

Recommended Frequency

Page, Phil. (2011). Thera-Band Exercises Effective for Piriformis Syndrome. See http://www.hygenicblog.com/2011/01/12/thera-band-exercises-effective-for-piriformis-syndrome/

Hamstring Curl (Seated)

Yass, Michael. (2015). The Pain Cure Rx: The Yass Method for Diagnosing and Resolving Chronic Pain. Hay House, Inc. p. 240.

Donkey Kicks

"Donkey Kicks with Flat Bands." See https://bodylastics.com/exercises/donkey-kicks-with-flat-resistance-bands/

Lateral Squat Walks with Resistance Band

Roberts, Anna Monette. (2012). "Squat Walk This Way: A Tush-Toning Thera-Band Exercise. See https://www.popsugar.com/fitness/Squat-Walks-Resistance-Band-22554623

Six Foam Rolling Moves to Conquer Back Pain

"How to Foam Roll Your Hamstrings." (2013). See https://www.youtube.com/watch?v=fMfe6DnlGvA.

Macdonald, G.Z., Button, D.C., Drinkwater, E.J., and Behm, D.G. (2014). "Foam Rolling as a Recovery Tool after an Intense Bout of Physical Activity." *Medicine & Science in Sports & Exercise* 46, no. 1, 131–142. doi: 10.1249/MSS.0b013e3182a123db.

Starrett, Kelly. (2015). *Becoming a Supple Leopard: The Ultimate Guide to Resolving Pain, Preventing Injury, and Optimizing Athletic Performance.* Victory Belt Publishing.

Three Foam Rolling Mistakes When Rolling Away Back Pain

"5 Foam Rolling Mistakes to Avoid." (2015). See http://fitness.mercola.com/sites/fitness/archive/2015/02/27/5-foam-rolling-mistakes.aspx.

Stull, Kyle. "Should You Foam Roll the Low Back?" See http://blog.nasm.org/ces/foam-roll-low-back/.

The Six-Minute Emergency Back Pain Treatment

Fanslau, Jill. (2016). "The Fit Man's Back-Saving Workout." See http://www.menshealth.com/fitness/exercises-to-prevent-back-pain?_ga=1.156404476.652772678.1492037609.

McKenzie, Robin A. (2011). *Treat Your Own Back.* Orthopedic Physical Therapy Products.

This One Simple Move Can Melt a Back Spasm in Just Five Minutes

"Static Back Knee Pillow Squeezes." See http://www.egoscue.com/WebMenus/ECiseHTML/453.html.

Sleep This Way

Alsaadi, S.M., McAuley, J.H., Hush, J.M., and Maher, C.G. (2011). "Prevalence of Sleep Disturbance in Patients with Low Back Pain." *European Spine Journal* 20, no. 5, 737–743. doi: 10.1007/s00586-010-1661-x.

"Back Pain? 5 Stretches to Do before Getting Out of Bed" (2013). See http://www.huffingtonpost.com/2012/05/08/back-pain-bed-stretches_n_1452898.html.

Gerhart, J.I., Burns, J.W., Post, K.M. et al. (2016). "Relationships Between Sleep Quality and Pain-Related Factors for People with Chronic Low Back Pain: Tests of Reciprocal and Time of Day Effects." Annals of Behavioral Medicine, 1–11. doi: 10.1007/s12160-016-9860-2

"How to Sleep with Lower Back Pain." See http://www.wikihow.com/Sleep-With-Lower-Back-Pain.

Jacobson, B.H., Boolani, A., Dunklee, G., Shepardson, A., and Acharya, H. (2010). "Effect of Prescribed Sleep Surfaces on Back Pain and Sleep Quality in Patients

Diagnosed with Low Back and Shoulder Pain." *Applied Ergonomics* 42, no. 1, 91–97. doi: 10.1016/j.apergo.2010.05.004.

"Pain and Sleep." See http://sleepfoundation.org/sleep-disorders-problems/pain-and-sleep.

Rodriguez, Diana. (2016). "Can Switching Your Sleep Position Ease Back Pain? See http://www.everydayhealth.com/news/switch-sleep-positions-ease-back-pain/.

"Sleeping Positions That Reduce Back Pain." See http://www.mayoclinic.org/diseases-conditions/back-pain/multimedia/sleeping-positions/sls-20076452.

"Sleeping with Back Pain." (2015). See http://www.webmd.com/back-pain/sleeping-positions-for-people-with-low-back-pain.

Resources

To fully take advantage of these back pain relief exercises, I highly recommend you get the following supplies.

Foam roller for self massage

> http://amzn.to/2ntTByb

Stretch strap

> http://amzn.to/2nGFwwF

Beginner set of resistance bands

> http://amzn.to/2ncfAw9

Theraband loops

> http://amzn.to/2nGs8Zt

Yoga mat

> http://amzn.to/2n1xOQF

Memory Foam Mattress for quality sleep

> http://amzn.to/2pkOsbi

About the Author

Since becoming a professional massage therapist in 2000, Morgan Sutherland has consistently helped thousands of clients manage their back pain with a combination of deep tissue work, cupping, and stretching. In 2002, he began a career-long tradition of continuing study by being trained in Tuina—the art of Chinese massage—at the world-famous Olympic Training Center in Beijing, China.

As an orthopedic massage therapist, Morgan specializes in treating chronic pain and sports injuries and helping restore proper range of motion. In 2006, Morgan became certified as a medical massage practitioner, giving him the knowledge and ability to work with physicians in a complementary healthcare partnership.

When he's not helping clients manage their back pain, he's writing blog posts about pain relief and self-care, in addition to teaching live and virtual workshops on how to incorporate massage cupping into a bodywork practice. Morgan has received the Angie's List Super Service Award for 2011, 2012, 2013, 2014, and 2015.

Morgan welcomes all comments about your real-life experiences implementing the stretches and exercises contained within this book. Thank you for reading.

Website: www.morganmassage.com

Email: morgan@morganmassage.com

Other Books by Morgan Sutherland, L.M.T.

21 Yoga Exercises For Lower Back Pain: Stretching Lower Back Pain Away With Yoga

Reverse Bad Posture Exercises: Fix Neck, Back & Shoulder Pain in Just 15 Minutes Per Day

Best Treatment for Sciatica Pain: Relieve Sciatica Symptoms, Piriformis Muscle Pain and SI Joint Pain in Just 15 Minutes Per Day

Resistance Band Workouts for Bad Posture and Back Pain: An Illustrated Resistance Band Exercise Book for Better Posture and Back Pain Relief

DIY Low Back Pain Relief: 9 Ways to Fix Low Back Pain So You Can Feel Like Yourself Again